About the Book

This book provides a unique summary of
international views on the developments that
are taking place in menopause research and
in the management of the menopausal syndrome.
It is based on the proceedings of the First
International Congress on the Menopause that
was held in France in June 1976. Leading clinicians
and research workers from over twenty different
countries took part in this important meeting
and together they tried, wherever possible, to
reach a consensus on the subjects under discussion.
The result was a stimulating and far-sighted
review of current knowledge.

The reports presented to the Congress by
the fourteen workshop chairmen are published
in this book. They cover almost all aspects of
menopause research and represent, insofar
as it is possible to do so, concise summaries
of the consensus reached on each subject area.
In addition, ten of the most important papers
presented at the meeting are also published
representing a cross section of the latest research
findings in this field.

Clinicians and research workers alike should
find this book an invaluable and entirely up-to-date
source of reference.

*Cover illustration from 'De Humani Corporis Fabrica'
by Andreas Vesalius.*

Consensus
on Menopause
Research

Consensus on Menopause Research

A Summary of International Opinion

Edited by P. A. van Keep
R. B. Greenblatt & M. Albeaux-Fernet

The Proceedings of the First International
Congress on the Menopause held at La Grande Motte,
France, in June, 1976, under the auspices of
The American Geriatric Society
and
The Medical Faculty of
The University of Montpellier

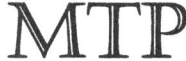

Published by MTP Press Limited,
St Leonard's House,
Lancaster,
England.

Copyright © 1976 MTP Press Limited.
Softcover reprint of the hardcover 1st edition 1976

ISBN 978-94-011-7181-6   ISBN 978-94-011-7179-3 (eBook)
DOI 10.1007/978-94-011-7179-3

Contents

Preface

This book contains a consensus on menopause research, a consensus reached during the First International Congress on the Menopause in June, 1976.

The Congress brought together about 165 people, most of whom are engaged in research in this field, in the resort town of La Grande Motte, near Montpellier, France. It was planned so that the main emphasis would be on the exchange of information in small Workshop sessions. Workshop Chairmen were asked to present summaries of their deliberations at the closing session. It is these summaries that form the essence of this text.

The Congress also included six Free Communications sessions. They are represented in this book by a small number of papers printed in full (selected from some 40 contributions in all) that in the opinion of the editors, contain data that particularly complement the Workshop summaries. All other papers are mentioned in these Proceedings by titles and by the name, affiliation and address of the first author.

Organizing this Congress was a stimulating and heart-warming experience. It was done by the staff of the International Health Foundation in Brussels and Geneva, under the considerate auspices of the American Geriatric Society and the Medical Faculty of the University of Montpellier. We are deeply grateful to these two bodies.

The organizers, who are also responsible for editing these Proceedings, would like to thank the many friends and colleagues who came to La Grande Motte to share their information and experiences, providing us with an exhaustive discussion of many facets of biological ageing in women. We are indebted to the chairmen of the Workshop and Free Communications sessions for the summaries and reports they made for us, and to all the people from the 22 countries represented who contributed time and talent to make this consensus possible.

The Congress was conceived by Prof. M. Albeaux-Fernet, France, who acted as Secretary-General. Prof. R. B. Greenblatt, USA, was Chairman of the Organization Committee; Dr. P. A. van Keep of the International Health Foundation, Belgium, was Programme Coordinator and Dr. M. Gelinet was Secretary for France.

P. A. van Keep

R. B. Greenblatt

M. Albeaux-Fernet

Section A

Consensus Reports by the Chairmen
of the Workshops

Editors' Note

In the Workshop Chairmen's reports that follow, where the Chairman is referring to a specific contribution made during the course of the workshop, he has usually indicated this by putting the name of the person responsible for that particular statement in brackets at the end of the appropriate sentence. Where, however, the report is referring to a published paper this is indicated by a reference number in the text and the full reference details are given at the end of the report in the normal way.

1

Workshop Report

The Climacteric Syndrome

Chairman : W. H. Utian

Groote Schuur Hospital and University of Cape Town, South Africa

Secretary: D. Serr

Tel-Aviv University Medical School, Israel

Introduction

There is an urgent need for a strict definition of the climacteric, the climacteric syndrome and the menopause. Without this definition no real progress can be made in assessing the extent of these conditions, their real effects and the efficacy of therapeutic procedures; nor can we appreciate what gaps in knowledge exist. Attitudes of despair prevailed until this century. It is only in recent years that a more enlightened approach can be noticed. Yet despite volumes that have been written, treating the problem from every aspect, no satisfactory definition has been found. Workers often have difficulty understanding each other's lines of research (Utian).

Definition and Symptoms

As a starting point it was proposed that the climacteric may be defined as 'a transitory phase in the human female between the ages of reproductive and non-reproductive ability'. The specific characteristics of this phase, clinical, metabolic, psycho-social and cross-cultural, must be taken into account. It is important to appreciate that 'menopause' refers only to cessation of menstruation and occurs during the climacteric phase. In defining the climacteric syndrome an attempt must be made to differentiate the true climacteric symptoms from those symptoms that are alleviated by hormone replacement therapy. Hauser was of the opinion that the occurrence of hot flushes was the only symptom specific to the climacteric.

Many attempts have been made to date the menopause, which is defined as the last menstrual period. Because of inaccurate recall by females as to the time of their last period, a median age should be determined at which 50% of females would have ceased menstruating, rather than the average age as is usually assessed. The median age for menopause is approximately 50–51, compared with an average of 47–48. The difference is accounted for by a tendency of women to understate their age at their last menstrual period. Based on this, there is no evidence to confirm suggestions that there has been any meaningful increase in the age at which menopause normally occurs (McKinlay).

There was a general feeling that hot flushes, perspiration and atrophic vaginitis are the only true early features of lack of estrogen, and that a different explanation must be sought to account for all the other symptoms usually attributed to 'estrogen deficiency' or listed as part of the climacteric syndrome (Utian).

Cross-cultural factors, apart from physical or psychological aspects, account for variations in symptomatology (See Report: Psycho-social Aspects). The concept of a 'psycho-somatic-socio-cultural' syndrome may well be proposed. A woman's assessment of cultural gains and losses affecting her way of life and social contacts contributes to the establishment of a state of 'well-being', a condition somewhere between happiness and worries. This assessment requires evaluation of such factors as fertility, menstruation, physical and emotional health, socio-personal aspects and marital relations (Maoz).

The doctor's attitude to symptom presentation is of fundamental importance (Serr). When the Kupperman Index is compared to plasma levels of FSH, LH and estradiol, no statistical correlation is found except in patients aged 30–35 years. The results suggest that the loss of cyclic activity in this group could result in elevation of gonadotrophins with accompanying disturbance of the autonomic nervous system. The absence of such a correlation might be accounted for by the fact that the Kupperman Index is non-specific (Abe).

Hot flushes and perspiration show a significant increase after castration. A similar increase in nervousness and tachycardia appears to exist, but does not reach significant levels (Punnonen).

There is a conflict and continuous interaction between person, organ and environment. Some symptoms occur before the menopause, some coinciding with it and others several years later (Hertz).

Symptoms may be divided into genital and extra-genital. It was suggested that a combined group of medical and para-medical workers should assess the contribution of each complaint to the climacteric syndrome and that an International Menopausal Index be derived so that comparative work can be accurately evaluated (Jaszmann).

Other symptomatology, e.g. bladder problems, could be estrogen-related (Studd, Foldes, Schleyer-Saunders).

Consequently such late symptomatology should be incorporated into the definition. The etiology of symptom formation can be listed as follows:

1. Hypothalamic–autonomic imbalance.
2. True estrogen deficiency,

   a) Early first signals: hot flushes, perspiration and atrophic vaginitis.
   b) Late consequences: related to metabolic changes in the end organ affected.

3. Psychological factors.
4. Socio-cultural factors.

Conclusions

A composite definition of climacteric, menopause and climacteric syndrome was derived.

- 1. The *climacteric* is that phase in the ageing process of women marking the transition from the reproductive stage of life to the non-reproductive stage.
2. *Menopause* indicates the final menstrual period and occurs during the climacteric. Present estimations date this at about 51 years.
3. The *climacteric* is sometimes, but not necessarily always, associated with symptomatology. When this occurs it may be termed the 'climacteric syndrome'.

   Climacteric symptoms and complaints are derived from three main components:

   a) Decreased ovarian activity with subsequent hormonal deficiency resulting in early symptoms (hot flushes, perspiration and atrophic vaginitis), and late symptoms related to the metabolic change in the end organ effected.

b) Socio-cultural, factors determined by the woman's environment.

c) Psychological factors, dependent on the structure of the woman's character.

The variety in symptomatology is the result of interaction between these three components.

The chairman emphasized in conclusion that future epidemiological and psycho-social studies into the effects of therapy should state precisely which component of the definition is being evaluated or treated.

Invited participants in the Workshop on The Climacteric Syndrome *were:*

T. Abe (*Japan*)   L. *Jaszmann* (*The Netherlands*)
M. Flint (*USA*)   B. *Maoz* (*Israel*)
J. J. Foldes (*Israel*)   S. M. *McKinlay* (*USA*)
G. A. Hauser (*Switzerland*)   R. Punnonen (*Finland*)
D. G. Hertz (*Israel*)   J. W. W. Studd (*UK*)

2

Workshop Report

Psycho-social Aspects of the Climacteric

Chairman : P. A. van Keep

The International Health Foundation, Brussels, Belgium

Secretary: M. Humphrey

St. George's Hospital Medical School, London, England

Introduction

At present about 5% of the world population are women between 45 and 54 years of age. They are on the threshold of the climacteric, a biological transformation, which certainly in Western society, coincides with considerable changes in a woman's life situation.

All changes, and particularly *the change*, require adaptation to the situation that follows (Hertz). Adaptation, however, is ideally an active process rather than a mere capitulation to the events. It was the nature of these changes and a woman's ability to adapt that were the themes of this workshop.

The effect that this biological transformation has on a woman's psyche and social situation is modified by many factors. An effort was made to define these factors and to determine their role. It was recognized, however, that these factors are strongly inter-related and that their influence is difficult to specify. The effects of ageing and the menopause have been studied with the aid of the Minnesota Multiphasic Personality Inventory (MMPI). Individual profiles were remarkably constant over five years, which suggests that the impact of the climacteric on a woman's personality is in no way dramatic (Krüskemper).

Psychological tests may be useful in identifying the woman who will have problems in going through the climacteric phase. They are also valuable in assessing the effects of hormone therapy (Fedor–Freybergh).

Cultural Influences

The influence of the culture in which a woman lives seems to be of overwhelming importance to the way in which she adjusts to the menopause. Some societies *reward* women in one way or another, for having reached the end of the fertile period. The significance of the menopause, and therefore its implication for health and behaviour, is different from that in societies that *punish* a woman for having reached the end of her youth.

A particularly striking illustration of this is the attitude of the Rahjput classes in India, who look forward to the menopause and experience few symptoms. This is because they emerge from Purdah at the end of their childbearing years, acquire higher status and can move around at will, freed from the 'dangerous contamination' of menstrual blood (Flint).

A similar situation was found in Israel. Arab women, for whom the end of the fertile period brings positive changes in their lives, were affected less by the menopause than researchers anticipated (Maoz).

It is clear that in Western society there is strong emphasis on youth and beauty. Cosmetics and even plastic surgery are part of the everyday lives of women in all age-groups, itself a reflection of the punitive attitude toward the menopause and ageing.

The severity of the climacteric syndrome, and particularly of its nervous symptoms, is different according to a number of pyschosocial co-ordinates. The woman who belongs to a lower socioeconomic group suffers more than the woman in a higher socioeconomic group. The availability of alternative roles, when children are still at home, for example, or when the woman has a meaningful job or is well-integrated into society, seems to be associated with an easier climacteric phase. In the lower socio-economic group, however, holding a job apparently has an adverse effect. This might be due to the nature of the work done, to the motivation to work or to the total burden that women in the lower socio-economic group bear in comparison with those who are better off and have greater 'manoeuvrability'.

The 'empty nest syndrome' is an attractive concept, but it is not a common cause of psychological disturbance. The distressed peri-menopausal woman who consults her doctor is most likely to have presented neurotic problems earlier in life as well. However, since the peri-menopause involves both biological and social loss, we ought to pay more attention to the predictive value of traumatic loss, such as the death of a parent in childhood. This is known to be associated with depression in adult life (Humphrey).

A late menarche is associated with fewer symptoms, and so is nulli-parity, higher income, having a child after forty, higher education and being unmarried (Jaszmann).

The impact of the climacteric on health seems to be stronger in urban than in rural populations; it is likely that to a large extent the differences may be accounted for by other than geographical factors (Schalaster).

Management

The doctor's attitude to his patient, an understanding of her specific difficulties and skill in counselling are of great importance in helping a woman through this phase of life (Kepes). The female doctor is perhaps more likely to fulfil these requirements than her male colleague. Women express their anxieties to female more freely than to male doctors, to whom they usually present only the somatic symptoms. It is understood that male doctors, particularly those trained in Balint methods, can overcome this apparent disadvantage (Weill–Hallé).

The initiative developed in France to help middle-aged women refresh their former professional abilities is to be applauded. The organization behind the programme, 'Re-travailler', concentrates on psychological conditioning to help women face professional life again.

Conclusions

A number of areas still need further study. These include the specific problems of single women (unmarried, divorced and widowed); the effects of therapy on social adaptation; the influence of the presence or absence of integration; the effect of nutrition and of sex-education; the influence of changes in society, values and beliefs on the climac-teric (syndrome); the influence of menopause on marital relations;

the attitude toward the menopause in different cultures (including the less technically-developed ones). But perhaps most important of all would be longitudinal studies with and without therapy. All these studies could help to determine the women who are least able to adapt and who could therefore be prone to go through a difficult phase.

It appears that education and information can help a woman live through the climacteric with a minimum of problems. Young people, understandably, show little interest. They are concerned with the more immediate problems of their reproductive lives. It seems more practical to inform the woman in her 40s about the true nature of these physical and psychological changes.

The psycho-social aspects of the menopause form an integral part of the picture and it is therefore misleading to look at the menopause and climacteric phase as purely biological phenomena.

Invited participants in the Workshop on Psycho-social Aspects of the Climacteric were:

P. Fedor-Freybergh (Sweden)
M. Flint (USA)
D. G. Hertz (Israel)
L. Jaszmann (The Netherlands)
S. Kepes (France)
G. Krüskemper (West Germany)

J. P. Mumford (The Netherlands)
U. Schalaster (West Germany)
L. Severne (Belgium)
A. Vagogne (France)
A. Vizzotto (Italy)
M. A. Weill-Hallé (France)

3

Releasing Factors in the Menopause

Chairman : W. D. Odell

UCLA-Harbor General Hospital Campus, California, USA

Secretary: M. L'Hermite

Hospital St. Pierre, Brussels, Belgium

There are extremely limited data available concerning concentrations, physiology and pathophysiology of gonadotrophin releasing factors in the menopause. One may summarize existing data as follows:

1. The concentrations in blood (and presumably secretion) of LH and FSH in menopausal women are pulsatile with cyclic variation at 10–20 min intervals.
2. In response to administration of the decapeptide LHRH (Luteinizing Hormone Releasing Hormone) to menopausal women, more LH is secreted than FSH when the two are stated in comparable terms, i.e., as increments above base line or in terms of the 2nd. IRP–HMG.
   Yet, during the basal menopausal state FSH concentrations are always higher than LH concentrations when stated in the same terms.
3. LHRH has been said to be present in larger amounts in blood of post-menopausal women than in eugonadal men or women.

It is worthwhile questioning (in view of number 2 above) whether elevated LH and FSH concentrations in the menopause stem solely from increased LHRH secretion. These data suggest the possibilities:

1. There is another polypeptide which predominately effects FSH secretion by the pituitary.

2. There is an alteration in the number of receptors on the pituitary cells that produce FSH. Therefore they have loss of sensitivity of LHRH.
3. There is an intrinsic property of the pituitary to secrete FSH autonomously in larger amounts of LH.

Conclusions

There appear to be several areas worthy of investigation in the relationship between LHRH, LH–FSH and ovarian physiology in the menopause. Studies should be done:

1. To determine whether the pulsatile LH and FSH secretion is related to pulsatile LHRH secretion.
2. To affirm or determine with improved techniques whether LHRH is in fact hypersecreted in the menopause.
3. To determine time and dose–response relationships between LH and FSH secretion and LHRH in the menopause.
4. To study the effects of ageing from peri-menopausal years to old age on the time and dose–response relationships described in the first paragraph (sub-section 3).

Invited participants in the Workshop on Releasing Factors in the Menopause *were:*

U. Gaspard *(Belgium)*   S. Matsumoto *(Japan)*
R. B. Greenblatt *(USA)*   A. Onnis *(Italy)*
H.-P. Klotz *(France)*   C. Robyn *(Belgium)*
V. B. Mahesh *(USA)*   D. Serr *(Israel)*

4

Gonadotrophins in the Menopause

Chairman : V. B. Mahesh

*Medical College of Georgia School of Medicine,
Augusta, Georgia, USA*

Review of Gonadotrophins Secretion

There is a dramatic elevation in blood levels of both FSH and LH in the menopause. Kohler and collaborators[1] found that the blood level of LH was elevated in spite of the fact there were no changes in its metabolic clearance rate. Coble and co-workers[2] found that the above was true for FSH as well. From these data, the mean production rate was calculated for FSH and LH in pre-menopausal and post-menopausal women. The mean increase of FSH in post-menopausal women was 14.1-fold over that found in the pre-menopausal state, while the increase in LH was 3.2-fold. This comparatively greater increase in FSH over LH results in FSH/LH ratios of > 1, whereas this ratio never exceeds 1 in the pre-menopausal state. These findings have been confirmed by several investigators.

The sequences of changes in steroids and gonadotrophins after cessation of menstruation have recently been compiled for a period up to 30 years by Chakravarti and co-workers. These investigators found a 13.4-fold elevation in FSH and a 3-fold elevation of LH within a year of the onset of menopause. After a further increase 2–3 years after onset, there was a gradual decline in both FSH and LH with age. The levels of both FSH and LH nevertheless were higher at all times (40–50% of maximum reached) as compared to the pre-menopausal years. Androstenedione, estrone and estradiol were reduced to approximately 20% of the early follicular phase level and showed only minor changes with time, if any at all. Serum testosterone, on the other hand, which was comparable with the early follicular phase levels in pre-menopausal years, declined by approximately 50% during the subsequent 4 years and then rose gradually with age.

In 1971 Adamopoulos and co-workers[3] reported that urinary gonadotrophins were elevated in the peri-menopausal years before the cessation of ovulatory function. A detailed study during the menopausal transition has been done recently by Sherman and co-workers[4]. The initial change appeared to be shorter cycles with a decrease primarily in the length of the follicular phase. This was accompanied by a decrease in the pre-ovulatory mid-cycle peak of estradiol, as well as lowered serum estradiol levels in the luteal phase. Serum LH during such cycles and serum progesterone during the luteal phase was comparable to that found in the normal menstrual cycle. In a few instances serum FSH was within normal limits, but in most of the cycles it was markedly elevated. In some cases there was a delayed maturation of the follicle, followed by ovulation in the presence of persistently high serum FSH and LH, with a diminished secretion of estrogens and progesterone. In others, vaginal bleeding occurred during a fall of serum estradiol with no associated rise or fall of progesterone.

Role of the Ovary in Menopause

There is an elevation in circulating gonadotrophins in gonadal dysgenesis, in premature ovarian failure and after ovariectomy in the human. In rats the post-castration changes occur as early as 8 hours after castration. Therefore, the most obvious explanation for elevated gonadotrophins in the post-menopause appeared to be the absence of the negative feed-back effect of ovarian steriods. Longcope[5] has demonstrated very low blood estradiol levels in post-menopausal women aged 50–90 years and a marked reduction in blood estrone. There appears to be no demonstrable change in blood levels of estradiol after ovariectomy in post-menopausal women, nor is there any increase after 3000 IU of HCG. This is in sharp contrast to the situation in men in the above age group, in whom HCG produces a marked response. Judd and collaborators[6] found only slightly higher estradiol levels in ovarian vein blood of post-menopausal women as compared to peripheral blood. However, testosterone was significantly elevated in ovarian vein blood of menopausal women when compared with that of normal women. There were also increases in androstenedione, albeit small. These findings were confirmed by Greenblatt and co-workers[7], who found the elevation in androstenedione greater than testosterone. Furthermore, after stimulation with 5000 IU of HCG, there was a dramatic increase in androstenedione and testosterone in ovarian vein blood with no change in estradiol. These findings confirm lowered steroid output of the ovary, particularly in estradiol secretion.

Why do the ovaries stop responding to gonadotrophins? Since ovarian estrogens are primarily produced by ovarian follicles, the belief that the menopause is due to follicular exhaustion is very popular. A quantitative morphological examination of the human follicular system by Block in 1952[8] revealed that, although there was a dramatic decline in the number of primordial follicles with age (a mean of 155 000 between the ages of 18–24 v. 8300 between 40–44), there were nevertheless a significant number of primordial follicles present at the onset of menopause. In 1970, in a study of 200 women above the age of 50 with abnormal bleeding, Novak reported evidence of a recent ovulation in 23%. In all post-menopausal ovaries studied there were a small number of primordial follicles with normal appearance and normal-looking ovum as determined by electron microscopic studies[9]. The explanation as to why these follicles do not respond to elevated gonadotrophins is not clear. In evaluating this lack of normal responsiveness, one must consider the data of Sherman and co-workers[4]. They found that during some cycles in the peri-menopausal period, delayed follicular maturation and corpus luteum function only occurred after persistently high endogenous FSH and LH levels over a long period of time, associated with a quantitative decrease in estrogen and progesterone secretion. An isolated case of pregnancy is reported in a peri-menopausal woman with high FSH and LH given 450 IU/day of a human menopausal gonadotrophin preparation. No systematic study of the response of the ovary to gonadotrophins during the peri-menopausal and early post-menopausal years has been reported thus far. A discussion of premature ovarian failure (premature menopause) indicated that the situation is somewhat different from normal menopause because here, according to most investigators, a complete exhaustion of ovarian follicles is found.

Is the lack of responsiveness of the post-menopausal ovary to gonadotrophins due to decreased receptors or to binding of gonado-trophins to the ovary? No systematic study has thus far appeared regarding the human ovary. Mills[10] has reported on his studies with rabbits that during a period of 4–6 hours before ovulation, the ovarian follicle does not respond to LH, even though there is no decrease in gonadotrophin binding. At this meeting Mori and co-workers reported a significant decrease in ovarian uptake of ^{125}I-HCG in old rats as compared to mature rats. In studies of this type one should consider not only the total binding, but also changes in binding due to changes in the quantity of various organelles in the ovary.

The question of a greater increase in FSH as compared to LH in the peri-menopause has been a subject of much discussion. The concept of an ovarian factor with negative feed-back on FSH—'inhibin' has been advanced, in view of a rising level of FSH in association with a decreasing number of ovarian follicles with age; the preferential suppression of LH over FSH with steroids; and high levels of FSH in peri-menopausal women as compared to pre-menopausal women with comparable blood steroid levels. There is evidence of the presence of such a factor in the testes as well.

Hypothalamic–Pituitary Feed-back System

The hypothalamic-pituitary axis in immaturity is very sensitive to the suppressive effect of sex steroids. At puberty there is a dramatic change in sensitivity and much larger quantities of steroids are re-quired to prevent the post-castration rise of gonadotrophins. Dilman postulates that his shift in sensitivity is progressive. In his experience, there is a period in the peri-menopause when urinary phenolsteroids and gonadotrophins are both elevated, indicating altered sensitivity of the hypothalamic–pituitary axis to steroids. After a period of compensation there is a breakdown of the system, leading to ovulatory failure. Dilman noted that changes in phenolsteroids did not corre-spond completely to identified estrogens. He thus postulated unknown compounds. Confirming Dilman's views somewhat, are Netter's observations[11] of high blood and urinary estradiol and serum FSH and LH in several menopausal patients. Sherman and co-workers[4] reported the contrary, noting a shorter follicular phase in peri-menopausal years with a decreased pre-ovulatory estrogen peak. The implication of their results is that the considerably lower estradiol levels

with a shorter length of exposure can trigger the surge of gonadotrophins, thus leading to ovulation.

The suppression of gonadotrophins with estrogens in peri-menopausal women is well-documented. No systematic and conclusive
comparisons have been done to evaluate the sensitivity of the hypothalamic–pituitary axis to such suppression. Reports presented at this
meeting by Gaspard and Robyn showed lowering of gonadotrophins—
both FSH and LH—in peri-menopausal women by doses of 20–25 µg
of ethinyl estradiol. These doses did not alter the FSH and LH level
in the luteal phase of the menstrual cycle and therefore they suggest
greater sensitivity to ethinyl estradiol in peri-menopausal women.
Although doses of 20–25 µg of ethinyl estradiol lowered gonadotrophins, doses as large as 50 µg were ineffective in restoring the
gonadotrophins to pre-menopausal levels, thus raising questions
regarding increased sensitivity. In 1968, Odell and co-workers[12]
showed that a dose of progesterone given to post-menopausal women
treated with estrogens induced an ovulatory-type surge of gonadotrophins. Wise et al.[13] found that a dose of 20 µg of ethinyl estradiol
followed by medroxyprogesterone acetate did not produce such a
surge, whereas the pre-treatment with 400 µg of ethinyl estradiol
induced it. Their work also suggests that higher doses of estrogens
than those used in oral contraceptive medication may be required to
suppress gonadotrophins to pre-menopausal levels. In our laboratory
an 8-fold higher dose of estradiol was necessary to prevent the post-
castration rise of gonadotrophins in 23-month-old anovulatory rats
as compared to young adult rats.

In studying the feed-back system around the menopause, attention
should also be given to thyroid function. Work by Cidlowski and
Muldoon[14] has shown that in the rat, thyroidectomy reduced estradiol
receptors in pituitary cytosol, whereas thyroid treatment increased
the number of these receptors proportionally to the dose administered.
Such an action of thyroid hormones is tissue-specific. Furthermore,
thyroid treatment or thyroidectomy alters the post-castration rise of
gonadotrophins and the pituitary's response to LH–RH (Mahesh).

The short loop feed-back mechanism also needs attention. Work by
Martini's group has shown that the administration of FSH to the rat
lowers pituitary FSH content and bio-assayable FSH-releasing
activity to the hypothalamus. Odell and co-workers[12] have reported
that LH administration in the rabbit lowers post-castration rise of
LH. Such a lowering is observed only up to 3 weeks after castration.

The pituitary responsiveness to LH–RH also deserves comment.

The work of most investigators has shown that the reponsiveness of the pituitary to LH–RH in the menopause is exaggerated. However, if one considers the pre-treatment levels and the percentage increment after LH–RH, the response appears to be similar to the pre-menopausal state. This is true for both FSH and LH and contrasts dramatically to the pre-pubertal state, in which the LH increment after LH–RH is much smaller.

The consensus was that the vasomotor symptoms in the climacteric phase are related more directly to estrogen decrease rather than gonadotrophin elevation. Worthy of mention is the fact that patients undergoing hypophysectomy for breast carcinoma do not show these symptoms. The reason for the lack of symptoms is not clear as both gonadotrophin and estrogen withdrawal occurs.

Some Current Theories of Cellular Ageing

In 1961 Hayflick and Moorhead[15] observed that normal diploid fibroblast cells have a finite ability to replicate *in vitro*. Subsequent work has shown that these population-doublings are inversely related to the age of the donor, and that the population-doubling of embryonic fibroblasts are directly related to the life-span of the donor species. In the ageing cell, the stoppage of proliferation is due either to a decrease in new DNA synthesis (G_1 block), or a block in the process of mitosis (G_2 block). These blocked or non-cycling cells remain in a non-proliferative stage until death or reversal of the procedure. Evidence of reversal of the non-proliferation process may be readily seen in the process of liver regeneration after injury or surgical removal of a part of the liver. Gelfant and Smith[16] suggest that the process of non-cycling cells is synonymous with cellular ageing and that this process is reversible. They propose that a study of factors that cause the non-cycling of cells and the reversal of this phenomenon during tissue regeneration may provide us with clues on the process of ageing.

Animal Models

One must be careful in extrapolating experimental data to humans because of species differences. Nevertheless, for a detailed study of hypothalamic–pituitary mechanisms and ovarian responsiveness, animal preparations are necessary. Furthermore the low cost, ready availability and the short life span between birth, cessation of ovarian function and death make them desirable. The ovary of the 23-month-old rat that has stopped ovulating for several months is atrophic and has few follicles. Nevertheless, when transplanted into castrated young females, cyclic ovulation takes place[17]. Epinephrine or levodopa administration results in the resumption of normal cycles in aged anovulatory rats. So does iproniazid, a drug that blocks the degradative metabolism of dopamine. Cyclicity is maintained only during the administration of the drug.

In the aged rat, the quantitative secretion of gonadotrophins is quite different as compared to the human. The pattern, however, is somewhat similar in as much as FSH increases very dramatically in comparison to LH, which is consistently low. The pituitary responds strikingly to LH–RH with massive and prolonged LH secretion (McPherson, Costoff and Mahesh). A hypothalamic cause is considered responsible for the cessation of ovulation. Ichinoe and collaborators reported during the session that the transplantation of ovaries of young mice into aged mice (C57 BL/6J strain) that had stopped ovulating resulted in cyclic ovulation, normal mating behaviour and pregnancy. The mouse of the CBA strain that lives for an average of 530 days displays virtually complete depletion of primary ovarian oocytes by 300–400 days of age.

The availability of rats and mice and their short life allow useful comparisons to be made with human mechanisms. They should be studied in an attempt to answer such questions as to why the ovarian follicle ceases to respond to gonadotrophins, and as to differences existing in hypothalamic–pituitary control mechanisms. The use of non-human primates should also be explored. Isolated reports indicate peri-menopausal and menopausal changes in rhesus monkeys between the ages of 25 and 30 years with a decrease in ovarian aromatase activity.

References

1. Kohler, P. O., Ross, G. T. and Odell, W. D. (1968). Metabolic clearance and production rates of human luteinizing hormone in pre and post-menopausal women. *J. Clin. Invest.*, **47**, 38
2. Coble, Y. D., Kohler, P. O., Cargille, C. M. and Ross, G. T. (1969). Production rates and metabolic clearance rates of human follicle-stimulating hormone in premenopausal and postmenopausal women. *J. Clin. Invest.*, **48**, 359
3. Adamopoulos, D. A., Loraine, J. A. and Dove, G. A. (1971). Endocrinological studies in women approaching the menopause. *J. Obstet. Gynaecol.*

4. Sherman, B. M., West, J. H. and Korenman, S. G. (1976). The menopausal transition: analysis of LH, FSH, estradiol, and progesterone concentrations during menstrual cycles of older women. *J. Clin. Endocrinol. Metab.*, **42**, 629

5. Longcope, C. (1971). Metabolic clearance rate and blood production rates of estrogens in post menopausal women. *Am. J. Obstet. Gynecol.*, **111**, 778

6. Judd, H. L., Judd, G. E., Lucas, W. E. and Yen, S. S. C. (1974). Endocrine functions of the postmenopausal ovary: concentration of androgens and estrogens in ovarian and peripheral vein blood. *J. Clin. Endocrinol. Metab.*, **39**, 1020

7. Greenblatt, R. B., Colle, M. L. and Mahesh, V. B. (1976). Ovarian and adrenal steroid production in postmenopausal women. *Obstet. Gynecol.*, **47**, 383

8. Block, E. (1952). Quantitative morphological investigation of the follicular system in women. *Acta Anat.*, **14**, 108

9. Costoff, A. and Mahesh, V. B. (1975). Primordial follicles with normal oocytes in the ovaries of postmenopausal women. *J. Am. Geriat. Soc.*, **23**, 193

10. Mills, T. M. and Savard, K. (1973). Steroidogenesis in ovarian follicles isolated from rabbits before and after mating. *Endocrinology*, **92**, 778

11. Netter, A. and Lambert, A. (1975). Etude hormonale préliminaire de la préménopause in la ménopause—Colloque Internationale de Biarritz of College de Gynecologie de Bordeaux et du Sud-Ouest (I. Bernard, M. Kollenc and A. Audebert, editors) pp. 28–37

12. Odell, W. D. and Swerdloff, R. S. (1968). Progestogen-induced luteinizing and follicle stimulating hormone surge in postmenopausal women: a stimulated ovulatory peak. *Proc. Nat. Acad. Sci.*, **61**, 529

13. Wise, A. J., Gross, M. A. and Schlach, D. S. (1973). Quantitative relationships of the pituitary-gonadal axis in postmenopausal women. *J. Lab. Clin. Med.*, **81**, 28

14. Cidlowski, J. A. and Muldoon, T. G. (1975). Modulation by thyroid hormones of cytoplasmic estrogen receptor concentrations in reproductive tissues of the rat. *Endocrinology*, **97**, 59

15. Hayflick, L. and Moorhead, P. S. (1961). The serial cultivation of human diploid cell strains. *Exp. Cell Res.*, **25**, 585

16. Gelfant, S. and Smith, J. G. (1972). Aging noncycling cells: an explanation. *Science*, **178**, 357

17. Peng, M. T. and Huang, H. H. (1972). Aging of hypothalamic-pituitary-ovarian function in the rat. *Fertil. Steril.*, **23**, 535

Invited participants in the Workshop on Gonadotrophins in the Menopause *were:*

S. K. Chakravarti (*UK*)
U. Gaspard (*Belgium*)
R. B. Greenblatt (*USA*)

C. Longcope (*USA*)
W. D. Odell (*USA*)
C. Robyn (*Belgium*)

5

Workshop Report

Prolactin and Menopause

Chairman : M. Ben-David

The Hebrew University, Hadassah Medical School, Jerusalem, Israel

Secretary: M. L'Hermite

Hospital St. Pierre, Brussels, Belgium

It was only five years ago that human prolactin was isolated, allowing the development of precise and sensitive assays, by means of which we could study its physiopathology. It should be pointed out that prolactin is not a single hormone, but in fact at least four isohormones[1]. The physiological significance of this phenomenon is as yet unknown. Although the roles of human prolactin in lactation was evident, it was also found to be present in relatively high amounts in the circulation of non-lactating women, as well as males and children. This fact, together with the recent discovery of the existence of membrane receptors for prolactin in a variety of tissues, including mammary glands, gonads, kidneys and liver, would indicate some role of prolactin in many physiological aspects other than lactation.

Prolactin and Ovarian Function

While prolactin was found to be essential for the maintenance of corpora lutea in many species, its role in the human menstrual cycle appears to be somewhat different. It seems that normal levels of circulating prolactin are not needed for the regulation of the normal menstrual cycle, since its suppression to subnormal levels throughout an entire menstrual cycle failed to induce any changes. However, *in vitro* human experiments suggested that a minimal priming with prolactin was essential for progesterone production by ovarian elements[2]. On the other hand, when serum prolactin levels are elevated, a serious interference with reproductive processes occurs, as manifested by luteal deficiency, and/or anovulation, leading to infertility and/or sterility[3]. Hyperprolactinaemia is not infrequent, and, furthermore, does not necessarily induce any galactorrhea, spontaneous or otherwise. Prolactin measurements are therefore advisable in any case of infertility to identify patients with unsuspected hyperprolactinaemic sterility syndrome. Anovulation in these cases is generally quite resistant to the classical treatments used for induction of ovulation, but can be cured very easily by suppression of hyperprolactinaemia by treatment with ergot derivatives such as 2Brα-ergocryptine methanesulfonate (bromocryptine = CB-154)[4].

The mechanisms by which hyperprolactinaemia interferes with the reproductive processes are still under investigation, although the data indicate that it could interfere both at ovarian and hypothalamo–pituitary levels[5]. Around the menopause, however, ovarian inactivity is not related to hyperprolactinaemia. On the contrary, the resulting low estrogen levels could be responsible for the lowered overall prolactin secretion[6].

Control of Prolactin Secretion

The hypothalamic control of prolactin secretion by the pituitary is mainly inhibitory. This is brought about by secretion of prolactin inhibiting factor (PIF) into the portal blood supply to the pituitary. Thyrotrophin-releasing hormone (TRH), which in pharmacological doses can release prolactin, does not seem to play any major physiological role in regulation of prolactin secretion. In conditions such as suckling and stress, the intervention of another hypothalamic factor that induces a prolactin release (PRF) is most likely needed. The secretion of PIF is activated by dopaminergic stimulation. Therefore either interference with dopamine synthesis (methyl-dopa) or storage (reserpine), or blockade of dopaminergic receptors (phenothiazines and butyrophenone-derivatives such as chlorpromazine, pimozide, halloperidol, etc.) will suppress PIF secretion and lead to hyperprolactinaemia. On the other hand, levo-dopa will increase PIF secretion and therefore decrease serum prolactin.

As far as pituitary responses of post-menopausal women to TRH, chlorpromazine and levo-dopa are concerned, the qualitative re-activity was found to be similar to that in reproductive-age women. However, standardization of these tests is awaited, especially with respect to the possible effects of ageing on quantitative reactivity. Also, the effect of stress on prolactin secretion, which is known to be an important stimulatory factor in women of reproductive age, has not yet been investigated in post-menopausal women.

Prolactin Interaction with Other Hormones

It should be emphasized that it is not yet determined whether elevation in circulating prolactin has any significance, e.g. in development of breast or endometrial cancer, in post-menopausal women. Furthermore, it is not known whether changes in circulating prolactin in combination with changes in other hormonal levels (such as of insulin, estrogens, thyroid hormones, corticosteroids, etc.) will especially affect the development of neoplasia. In this respect, not only are blood levels involved, but reports have appeared recently of changes in the number of receptors in the target organs. An example of the complexity of the inter-relationships can be found in the prevention of lactation by estrogens. Lactation can be prevented both by suppression of immediate post-partum prolactin secretion and by administration of high doses of estrogens, although these will lead to still greater prolactin concentrations. It was found that in both cases (either of suppressed prolactin secretion alone or increased prolactin secretion together with high estrogen levels), the production of kappa–casein (one of the specific constituents of milk) was suppressed. Hence the mechanism by which high estrogen levels may prevent lactation resides apparently in a direct action on the mammary gland itself, probably at a point beyond the stimulation of specific enzymatic activities by prolactin. Therefore it would be preferable to prevent post-partum lactation with the use of prolactin suppressors such as CB–154 rather than with estrogens or other means.

Estrogens and Prolactin

There are, indeed, indirect as well as direct arguments to indicate a relationship between estrogens and prolactin secretion[7]. It appears that basal prolactin secretion does not change much with age in males. In women, it increases after puberty and decreases after menopause.

These changes are parallel to estrogenic secretion. Other indirect indications of this inter-relationship reside in:

1. The parallelism between progressively increased estrogens and prolactin secretion during pregnancy.
2. The tendency towards occurrence of midcycle and luteal phase increased prolactin concentrations.

The relationship is further supported by increases in circulating prolactin after administration of pharmacological doses of non-natural estrogenic compounds in cycling as well as post-menopausal women.

Indeed the oral administration of 25 μg ethinylestradiol per day to post-menopausal women resulted within a few days in a 2.5-fold increase in basal prolactin levels, which were thus slightly higher than the average normal level encountered in women of reproductive age[7]. It appears, however, that pituitary prolactin reactivity to exogenous estrogens is greater in post-menopausal women with low endogenous estrogens and prolactin secretions than in normally cycling women. The elucidation of this phenomenon needs further investigation.

Nevertheless, the oral administration of natural conjugated estrogens in doses usually sufficient to eliminate objective as well as subjective menopausal symptoms (hot flushes, osteoporosis, etc.), did not result in any elevation of prolactin concentration.

The oral administration of 1.25 mg of natural conjugated estrogens failed thus to increase prolactin. Higher doses, however, have not yet been tested in post-menopausal women, although they are only seldom needed. It appears that natural conjugated estrogens in doses which are sufficient for treatment of the menopausal syndrome, but which do not affect prolactin secretion, should be preferred to the presently available synthetic estrogenic compounds, for which the treatment and prolactin-stimulatory doses are similar.

Additional hormonal treatments have been used and/or proposed in menopause therapy, such as the combination of androgens with estrogens, cyclic addition of progestagens to estrogens, etc. The possible effects of such regimens upon prolactin secretion have not yet been investigated in the post-menopausal state.

The true incidence of prolactin-secreting pituitary adenomas in post-menopausal women is not yet documented. As in younger women, the administration of estrogens to subjects having a pre-existing pituitary adenoma might be risky[5]. The use of natural estrogens, which do not seem to exert any major effect on prolactin secretion in normal post-menopausal women, should be recommended.

Nevertheless, prolactin determination may be advisable before initiating long-term estrogenic treatment, in order to avoid the possibility of hyperprolactinaemia. Perhaps, too, a follow-up of prolactin should also be recommended at regular (yearly?) intervals in the course of such treatment.

Conclusions

In women prolactin increases after puberty and decreases after menopause. These changes appear to be parallel to estrogenic secretion.

While in reproductive-age women consistent hyperprolactinaemia may abolish ovarian responsiveness to gonadotrophins, ovarian inactivity in the menopause is not related to hyperprolactinaemia. During the menopause, in contrast to synthetic estrogens, the natural estrogens in doses usually sufficient to eliminate post-menopausal symptoms (hot flushes, osteoporosis, etc.) do not elevate serum prolactin. Therefore, as far as prolactin elevation is concerned, when estrogen therapy is needed in the menopause the use of natural estrogens should be preferred.

The possible effects of additional hormonal treatments on prolactin secretion, for example a combination of androgens and estrogens or cyclic addition of progesterones to estrogens, have not yet been investigated in the post-menopausal state.

Finally, it is not yet known with confidence whether elevation in circulating prolactin (either alone or in conjunction with changes of other hormones, such as insulin, estrogens, thyroid hormones, corticosteroids, etc.) has any significance in connection with the development of breast or endometrial cancer or other neoplasia in the menopausal state.

References

1. Ben-David, M. and Chrambach, A. (1974). Isolation of human prolactin *isohormones* from amniotic fluid. *Endocr. Res. Commun.*, **1**, 193
2. McNatty, K. P., Sawers, R. S. and McNeilly, A. S. (1974). A possible role of prolactin in the control of steroid secretion by the human Graafian follicle. *Nature (London)*, **250**, 653
3. Yarkoni, S., Polishuk, W. Z., Spitz, I. M. and Ben-David, M. (1976). Inhibitory effect of hyperprolactinemia on induction of ovulation by gonadotropins. *J. Clin. Endocr. Metab.* (submitted for publication)

4. Thorner, M. O., McNeilly, A. S., Hagan, C. and Besser, G. M. (1974). Long term treatment of galactorrhoea and hypogonadism with bromocriptine. *Br. Med. J.*, **2**, 419
5. L'Hermite, M., Caufriez, A., Vekemans, M., Denayer, P. and Robyn, C. (1976). Pharmacological and pathological aspects of human prolactin secretion. In: *Clinical Reproductive Neuroendocrinology* (P. O. Hubinont, M. L'Hermite and C. Robyn, editors) (Basel, S. Karger)
6. Vekemans, M. and Robyn, C. (1975). Influence of age on serum prolactin in women and men. *Br. Med. J.*, **4**, 738
7. Robyn, C., Delvoye, P., van Exter, C., Vekemans, M., Caufriez, A., Denayer, P., Delogne-Desnoeck, J. and L'Hermite, M. (1976). Physiological and pharmacological factors influencing prolactin secretion and their relation to human reproduction. In: *Prolactin and Human Reproduction* (P. G. Crosignani and C. Robyn, editors) (London and New York, Academic Press)

Invited participants in the Workshop on Prolactin and Menopause *were:*

P. G. Crosignani (Italy)	*P. Kicovic (The Netherlands)*
R. D. Gambrell Jr. (USA)	*V. B. Mahesh (USA)*
U. Gaspard (Belgium)	*W. D. Odell (USA)*
S. Geller (France)	*C. Robyn (Belgium)*
R. B. Greenblatt (USA)	*R. Wenner (Switzerland)*

6

Workshop Report

Post-menopausal Estrogen Production

Chairman : J. H. H. Thijssen

Academisch Ziekenhuis Utrecht, Utrecht, The Netherlands

Secretary: C. Longcope

Worcester Foundation for Experimental Biology, Shrewsbury, Massachusetts, USA

The Pre-menopause

Before the menopause the main source of estradiol is direct secretion by the ovaries. Over 90% of estradiol comes from this source. About 50% of estrone results from secretion by the ovary, the remainder originates from the peripheral conversion of androstenedione to estrone and from estradiol to estrone. Substantial amounts of androstenedione are secreted by the ovaries and adrenals, with larger contributions coming from the adrenals.

Of the testosterone production, 60–70% arises from the peripheral conversion of androstenedione to testosterone, with some secretion by ovaries and adrenals.

The Peri-menopausal Period

Data on actual hormone secretion by the ovaries during the peri-menopausal years are lacking, although there appears to be a gradual alteration in the steroid secretory pattern of the ovary. Plasma levels of estrogens and of androgens appear to decline slowly during those years. In the first 3 years following the cessation of menstruation this decline seems to continue.

The Post-menopause

Data discussed in the ensuing paragraphs are gathered from studies of women more than two years after their menopause.

Plasma Levels

From the data presented, it appears that plasma levels remain stable. For estrone, mean values range from 20–40 pg/ml, and for estradiol from 9–15 pg/ml. Urinary excretion of estrone and estriol also remains stable. There seems to be a small decrease in estrogen activity as measured by urinary sediment cytology. The reason for this discrepancy remains to be elucidated.

Plasma androstenedione levels remain stable at 0.6–0.9 ng/ml, while testosterone levels range from 0.2–0.3 ng/ml. There appears to be some fluctuation in the testosterone level in relation to age, changes that are statistically significant, but of doubtful physiological significance.

Blood Production Rates

The metabolic clearance rates of both androgens and estrogens are slightly lower in post-menopausal women. A decrease by 10–20% compared to pre-menopausal women was observed. Until the age of 75, there apparently is no decline in the clearance rates of either androgens or estrogens. Therefore the blood production rates, calculated from the plasma levels and the metabolic clearance rates, remain essentially unchanged from two years after the menopause.

The blood production rate for estrone amounts to about 40 μg/day, for estradiol about 10 μg/day, for androstenedione 1.5 μg/day and testosterone about 150 μg/day.

Biogenesis of Estrogens

Estrogens in post-menopausal women originate almost completely from the so-called peripheral conversion of androgens to estrogens. Due to inherent errors in the methodology used, a minimal contribution from direct secretion by the ovaries and/or adrenals cannot be excluded in all women. Discounting very obese women the fractional conversion rate of androstenedione to estrone rises from a pre-menopausal mean of 0.015 to a post-menopausal mean of 0.025. It appears that the major determinant is the menopausal status rather than the age of the woman as such. In the groups studied, where maximal weight was less than 90 kg, a correlation between the fractional conversion rate and body weight could not be demonstrated. The reason for the increased conversion rate after the menopause remains obscure.

Steroid Secretion by the Ovaries

Regarding androgen secretion after the menopause, all data point to the fact that the ovary continues to secrete androstenedione and testosterone. Available data indicate that the post-menopausal ovary contributes directly and indirectly to about 50% of the testosterone production. About a third of androstenedione production originates in the ovaries. Of interest is the increased secretion of testosterone by the post-menopausal ovary. While the acute administration of huge amounts of human HCG seems to stimulate ovarian androgen secretion, it does not appear to have any effect on estradiol levels.

Conclusions

The ovaries of women more than two years after their menopause secrete substantial amounts of androgens, but insignificant quantities of estrogens. Estrone becomes the major circulating free estrogen. It arises almost entirely from the peripheral conversion of androstene-dione. Although knowledge concerning the production of sex steroids has increased markedly in recent years, certain aspects remain unknown.

There is a question about factors influencing the peripheral conversion of androgens to estrogen. It is also unclear, firstly, whether there is another stimulus to adrenal androgen production other than ACTH, and secondly, why, when estrogen production appears to remain relatively stable after the menopause, there is a gradual decline in the biological effects of estrogen as manifested by vaginal cytology.

References

1. Greenblatt, R. B., Colle, F. M. L. and Mahesh, V. (1976). Ovarian and adrenal steroid production in the postmenopausal woman. *Obstet. Gynecol.*, **47**, 383
2. Hensell, D. L., Grodin, J. M., Brennet, P. F., Siiteri, P. F. and MacDonald, P. C. (1974). Plasma precursors of estrogens. II. Correlation of the extent of conversion of plasma androstenedione to estrone with age. *J. Clin. Endocrinol. Metab.*, **38**, 476
3. Judd, H. L., Judd, G. E., Lucas, W. E. and Yen, S. S. C. (1974). Endocrine function of the postmenopausal ovary: concentration of androgens and estrogens in ovarian and peripheral vein blood. *J. Clin. Endocrinol. Metab.*, **39**, 1020
4. Longcope, C. (1971). Metabolic clearance and blood production rates of estrogens in postmenopausal women. *Am. J. Obstet. Gynecol.*, **111**, 778
5. Poortman, J., Thijssen, J. H. H. and Schwarz, F. (1973). Androgen production and conversion to estrogens in normal postmenopausal women and in selected breast cancer patients. *J. Clin. Endocrinol. Metab.*, **37**, 101
6. Vermeulen, A. (1976). The hormonal activity of the postmenopausal ovary. *J. Clin. Endocrinol. Metab.*, **42**, 247

Invited participants in the Workshop on Post-menopausal Estrogen Production *were:*

P. Kemeter (*Austria*)
P. Kicovic (*The Netherlands*)
V. B. Mahesh (*USA*)
I. Mori (*Japan*)

B. E. C. Nordin (*UK*)
S. Takenaka (*Japan*)
L. Tax (*The Netherlands*)

7

Genital Organs in the Menopause

Chairman : R. J. Beard

Royal Sussex County Hospital, Brighton, England

The changes that occur in the genital organs at the menopause were discussed with particular reference to the effects of estrogen deficiency and replacement therapy. The organs discussed were as follows: vulva, vagina, cervix, uterus and ovaries.

Vulva

Vulva skin undergoes atrophy as part of general ageing, along with skin in other sites. However, the atrophy may be greater here and more specifically related to estrogen deficiency than at other sites of the body. Vulval dystrophies and pruritus are much more common in post-menopausal women. Unfortunately there are no data to show that these conditions are caused specifically by estrogen deficiency, but suffice it to say that these conditions may be greatly improved by estrogen and corticosteroid therapy. The corticosteroid should not be too strong because it usually has to be given for a long period of time. Dienestrol cream and 1% hydrocortisone cream mixed in equal parts was mentioned as a useful therapy (Beard). It is important that all local infections are treated adequately with locally-active fungicides and broad spectrum antibiotics.

Vagina

Atrophy of vaginal skin in post-menopausal women *is* directly related to estrogen deficiency. The clinical problems thus produced include atrophic vaginitis and dyspareunia due to vaginal dryness and shrinkage. These problems are often worse where the woman has not had a vaginal delivery or if intercourse is infrequent, or resumed after a long time. These problems can always be prevented by estrogen therapy. Several of the participants prescribed estrogen cream when the symptom continued despite oral therapy or when systemic administration was contraindicated. Several instances of the systemic absorption of estrogen from the vagina were described, however very little is known about this. Further research would be welcomed, because one often uses local estrogens when systemic administration is contra-indicated.

When a woman has not had intercourse before the menopause or marries again after a long abstinence it is most important that she is given adequate estrogen therapy. This is especially true for the former, where in addition the use of dilators or reverse perineorrhaphy may be required. On the other hand, this shrinkage of the vagina may help the vaginal laxity that may occur after this age. This might be the only natural benefit to result from the menopause.

The kariopyknotic index and maturation percentage is of limited value in the management of the patients. Cross-sectional studies show poor correlation; but in any individual there is a reasonably high correlation with the estrogen status and response to treatment especially if the cytology is performed serially. Among the many parameters measured using 1 mg norgestrel and 1.25 mg of conjugated estrogens with controls, it was interesting to note that vasomotor symptoms were improved equally by both hormones, while it was only conjugated estrogens that improved the maturation index.

Cervix

The squamo-columnar junction usually retreats into the endocervical canal. In young women the increased estrogen levels during pregnancy and oral contraception lead to the opposite, but there is no evidence of an increase in erosions in estrogen-treated post-menopausal women. Mucus—produced from the endocervical canal—is definitely increased. Some workers believe the incidence of benign endocervical polyps increases too (Schneider), while others take the contrary view (Beard).

Uterus

The uterus becomes atrophied. Fibroids often do the same and become calcified. Estrogen therapy limits this atrophy and may enlarge fibroids very suddenly. Two such cases observed recently were reported, one needing an emergency laparotomy and hysterectomy because of ruptured veins on the surface of the enlarged fibroids (Beard).

The detection and management of endometrial abnormalities is regarded as important. Some prefer an endometrial biopsy with the Vabra or Karman-type suction uterine curettes rather than the jet washer. The importance of checking patency of the endocervical canal with a fine uterine sound before starting estrogen therapy was stressed (Casey, Schneider).

Ovaries

The ovary diminishes in size from the age of 30 and the rate accelerates after the age of 60. The number of functional cysts increases with age to maximum at 40–45 years. Histochemical staining shows an increase in lipid deposition and changes in the walls of vessels (Matsumoto).

There is no evidence that estrogen therapy affects the incidence of ovarian malignancy. The difficulty of diagnosis and the high mortality of ovarian malignancies are regarded as major problems. This risk of malignancy of the ovaries should, according to some participants (Casey, Schneider), encourage early removal of ovaries. Others, especially the English and Japanese, were more conservative. They felt that the risk of malignancy is outweighed by the benefits of small hormonal contribution from the post-menopausal ovary (Cooke).

After the menopause no latent follicular activity can be stimulated by massive doses of gonadotrophins (Ichinoe).

Invited participants in the Workshop on Genital Organs in the Menopause *were:*

M. J. Casey (*USA*)   K. Ichinoe (*Japan*)
A. C. Comninos (*Greece*)   S. Matsumoto (*Japan*)
I. D. Cooke (*UK*)   G. T. Schneider (*USA*)

8

Non-genital Target Tissues of Estrogens

Chairman : L. Rauramo

The University Central Hospital of Turku, Turku, Finland

Secretary: H. Kopera

University of Graz, Graz, Austria

Estrogens and the Urinary Tract

Estrogen deficiency causes atrophic changes of the urethra and bladder in a very high percentage of post-menopausal women. The consequences are atrophic cystitis, urethritis, ectropion urethrae, kolpitis, bacterial and fungal infections, loss of tonus of the bladder and urinary incontinence.

These pathological conditions improve or can be cured in the majority of cases by local or systemic estrogen substitution therapy (Lauritzen). It was emphasized that it is not only atrophy and its sequelae that react well to estrogen treatment. So do urethral ectropion, which is curable in nearly every case; and first-degree urinary stress incontinence (urge incontinence), where improvement in 90% and cure in about 80% of cases can be obtained. On the other hand, real stress incontinence, which is due to insufficiency of the sphincter, often responds better to surgery (Schleyer–Saunders). Administration of estrogens for the prophylaxis and treatment of urinary tract diseases in post-menopausal women is to be recommended.

Estrogens and the Psyche

The theory that estrogens can influence human behaviour and

modify, or even determine, specific psychic functions is wide-spread and hardly disputed. There are, however, few well-designed experiments and unquestionable results to support it. Although convincing experimental data are increasing, it must be remembered that the theory is still not proved. Research workers using animals are undoubtedly better off. They face simpler, but by no means simple, problems and have fewer difficulties in performing controlled studies. Hence their output of work is considerable. The complex influences of estrogens on human psychic functions, however, are much less readily definable, and are still far from being elucidated, even though our knowledge has been enriched by:

1. Careful observations of patients with abnormally low or high estrogen concentrations.
2. Studies of certain aspects of neurological and psychological functions in correlation with periodical changes in the menstrual cycle or estrogen therapy.

It would seem that at mid-cycle general activity increases and performance improves, but the changes are possibly too small to prove a physiological rhythm in the working capacity of women. Certain objective effects are better documented. They include an influence on general well-being and affective state as well as on cyclic fluctuations of emotionality, fatigue and irritability. A connection also appears to exist with psychodynamic changes.

Estrogens in physiological quantities do not appear to modify or impair libido and human sexual behaviour, although sex hormones are essential for the maintenance and control of their intensity. High doses of estrogens, in general decrease sexual desire and potency, besides causing mood changes and evoking functional autonomic symptoms (Kopera).

The question as to whether estrogens exert an influence upon mental functioning demonstrated by means of psychometric tests, is still insufficiently investigated. The evidence that estrogens slow or stop the gradual psychological downhill trend in ageing women (Kantor, Michael and Shore[1]) is less convincing after about 1 year of treatment. Rauramo and his colleagues performed a number of psychological tests and psychometric measurements on 65 ovariectomized and hysterectomized patients, some of whom were treated with estrogens. A comparison was made with a hysterectomized control group. The results did not show any difference in cognitive or attentive variables, but it did seem that emotional variables were affected by estrogen administration. Subjects not receiving estrogens clearly felt impairment of memory, of attention and the ability to concentrate, although psychometric tests failed to show this.

A similar influence of estrogens is also suggested by results of an investigation done with the MMPI (Minnesota Multiphasic Personality Inventory) on 165 women seeking medical advice to reduce excessive body weight. Pre-menopausal women were found to be psychologically more stable than post-menopausal patients (G. Krüskemper). Significant effects of estrogen therapy on a number of psychological tests were reported by van Hulle and Demol who performed a double-blind study on post-menopausal women.

Obviously trials with psychometric tests indicate possible effects of estrogens on mental functioning, yet the available data are still insufficient for final conclusions.

Estrogens and the Skin

The thickness of the epidermis and the number of mitoses decrease sharply after castration. Pathological deterioration can be significantly prevented or reduced with estrogen therapy (Rauramo, Punnonen).

Reports of other investigators confirmed that estrogens, at least in some patients, favourably affect both elasticity and colour of the hair. A beneficial influence of estrogens on the skin could still be found after three years of treatment. Similar encouraging results of estrogen therapy on the skin, indicating increased protein synthesis, were observed in studies done by Aertgeerts[2]. Reference was also made to Prijot's results[3] using oral estriol in the treatment of keratoconjunctivitis sicca, in which 16 out of 24 patients were cured and improvement was obtained in a further 3. Positive effects of estrogens on seborrhoea and acne were reported by various participants. Estrogens unquestionably influence the skin by preventing epidermal atrophy and reduced mitosis after estrogen deficiency by inducing extracellular water retention, stimulating hyaluronidase, improving skin circulation and affecting hair follicles and sebum production.

Estrogen and Growth Hormone, Insulin Secretion and Blood Glucose

Five years after menopause, glucose and serum immuno-reactive insulin (IRI) response to tolbutamide are not impaired. Hence menopause does not cause disturbance of carbohydrate metabolism in women without a disposition to diabetes. Even obese women showed a normal glucose and IRI-response. Moreover, 3–7 years' administration of natural estrogens in the post-menopause has no diabetogenic effect in obese or non-obese women. The growth hormone secretory capacity (rather low in all subjects studied) was found to be slightly higher in post-menopausal women under estrogen therapy than in matched controls (Rauramo, Syvälahti, Erkkola and Punnonen).

Estrogen and Thyroid Function

The physiological influences of ovarian hormones on the thyroid have long been known. They include transient swelling of the thyroid gland, changes in basal metabolism and of serum-iodine levels during the menstrual period. Effects of ovariectomy and estrogen administration have also been reported.

The thyroid gland enlarges during pregnancy, although its function is apparently not severely altered. In 1948 an elevation of the protein-bound iodine level in pregnancy was discovered. It appears to be a physiological reaction without signs of hyperthyroidism. A similar rise in PBI was found in 1952 after estrogen administration in non-pregnant subjects. Research workers subsequently described an increased ability of the thyroxine binding serum protein (TBP or TBG) to bind thyroxine as a consequence of estrogen treatment or pregnancy. Current information suggests that estrogens—mainly in pharmacological doses—can influence thyroid hormone economy through the following mechanisms:

1. An increase in the thyroxine-binding capacity of serum as part of a general effect on transport proteins. This seems to be the primary effect of estrogens. It is regularly seen in women under therapy with contraceptive preparations containing higher concentrations of estrogens. It can be a quantitative increase in TBG—which is more likely—or an increase in the binding sites per protein molecule.

2. An increase in the concentration of PBI or serum T_4, a secondary effect to the one mentioned above. It is accompanied by effects on the peripheral metabolism of T_4, a proportionate decrease in its fractional turnover rate with the result that daily T_4 disposal is unchanged.

3. An increase of thyroid function (uptake of radioiodide and/or hormone release rate). It is only seen in infants treated with large doses of estrogens and in a mild form in pregnancy.
4. Acute suppressive effects on the secretion of thyroid stimulating hormone and—in high doses—on thyroid release which are not mediated by TBG, total thyroxine, free thyroxine or cortisol.

Age, the estrogenic compound, dosage and duration of treatment appear to be the important determinants of the thyroidal effects of estrogen in humans (Kopera).

Thyroid function does not change in puberty or as a consequence of menopause. However, changes which are not sex-related do occur as a consequence of ageing. Thus TBG decreases until the age of 40 and thereafter increases again. Whereas T_4 concentration remains more or less unchanged with increasing age, T_3 steadily declines. A natural yearly loss of 0.8 ng T_3 in serum concentration has been calculated (H. L. Krüskemper). It was concluded that estrogens exert but a weak influence upon thyroid function in physiological concentrations.

Conclusions

The workshop concluded that the effects of estrogens have not been studied adequately on all non-genital target organs. More work complying with the principal requirements of clinical pharmacologic trials should be done to elucidate the influence of estrogens on psychic functions, on the skin, on the eye and on blood circulation.

References

1. Kator, H. I., Michael, C. M. and Shore, H. (1973). Estrogen for older women. *Am. J. Obstet. Gynecol.*, **116**, 115.
2. Aertgeerts, J. (1972). Influence d'une traitement oestrogène sur la peau de femmes ménopausées ou castrées. *Brux.-Méd.*, **3**, 215
3. Prijot, E., Barzin, L. and Destexhe, B. (1972). Essai de traitement hormonal de la kérato-conjunctivite sèche. *Bull. Soc. Belge Ophtal.*, **162**, 795

Invited participants in the Workshop on Non-genital Target Tissues of Estrogens *were:*

A. C. Comninos *(Greece)* Ch. Lauritzen *(West Germany)*
R. Demol *(Belgium)* J. Mirouze *(France)*
R. Klapper *(USA)* R. Punnonen *(Finland)*
G. Krüskemper *(West Germany)* E. Schleyer-Saunders *(UK)*
H. L. Krüskemper *(West Germany)* G. Weiland *(West Germany)*

9

The Estrogen Deficiency Syndrome and the Management of the Patient

Chairman : Ch. Lauritzen

Universität Ulm, Ulm/Donau, West Germany

The menopause and the climacteric are the consequences of ageing of the ovaries. These organs are the only endocrine glands that cease to function long before the end of life, in most cases after about 50 years of age.

This ovarian insufficiency results in estrogen deficiency with its attendant problems. Endocrine-metabolic studies suggest now that a substitute for the missing hormones ought to be considered.

Definition

The estrogen-deficiency syndrome is defined as a complex of typical, but by no means specific symptoms which are mostly of autonomous hypothalamic origin. These subjective climacteric complaints are experienced either as vasomotor, neurodystonic or psychic disturbances. They are apparently caused by the process of a relative decrease of estrogen in the *target tissues*, rather than by a fall in the absolute level.

The estrogen-deficiency syndrome also includes metabolic alterations and atrophic changes of the urogenital tract. All these symptoms are caused by the decrease of estrogens below a threshold level and may be ameliorated or even disappear altogether if these hormones are replaced.

Justification of Treatment

Climacteric complaints can cause a woman much physical, emotional and even social hardship. Therefore the decreasing estrogen level is a primary justification for estrogen replacement. It was agreed that the climacteric process can not be regarded as 'natural' or 'physiologic' if it is associated with debilitating complaints, and that the borderline between the physiological and the pathological is crossed when symptoms become complaints and the patient is obviously suffering as a result. The same holds in the case of a woman who experiences organic lesions due to estrogen deficiency.

Indications for Estrogen Therapy

There should always be a clear indication for estrogen therapy. The indiscriminate use of hormone replacement therapy is to be avoided. Whether or not treatment is indicated depends on the symptoms the patient presents, on the number and severity of the complaints and on the way in which she reacts. Certainly a woman ought to be treated if she goes to her doctor with climacteric problems and specifically asks for help. Estrogen therapy should not be considered without the consent and full co-operation of the patient, and no patient should be persuaded to undergo it. Once begun, the patient should be kept informed of all aspects of the treatment. Atrophic changes of the vulva, vagina, urethra and bladder, or signs of beginning osteoporosis, are clear indications for estrogen therapy. There is, however, a strong point to be made for prophylactic treatment. It seems logical to prevent the symptoms of the deficiency syndrome rather than to treat them when they occur.

Who Should be Treated Preventatively?

It would be highly desirable to have better criteria in order to establish who really needs estrogen therapy and who does not. At present, certainly, there is no way of predicting who will suffer from a severe estrogen deficiency syndrome. Assessment of the degree of proliferation from vaginal smears and determination of estrogens in blood and urine will only provide the estrogen status at a given time. No one can predict how these values might develop. So at present the criteria for deciding who should receive preventive therapy are more often subjective rather than objective.

Undeniable candidates for full preventive substitution are early-castrated women, the woman with an atrophic smear together with climacteric complaints, and the woman with signs of beginning osteoporosis. Arguments can be produced for prophylactic treatment of a greater part of the population. In practice, however, most patients will begin estrogen therapy only at the time when they go to the doctor with metrorrhagia, hot flushes or atrophic vaginitis. Even in these cases it is not too late to start estrogen therapy, not only to cure the symptoms present, but also to prevent later consequences of the estrogen-deficiency syndrome.

How Long Should Treatment be Given?

There are two schools of thought on this. The first is that only severe symptoms should be treated, and with the smallest possible doses for the shortest possible time. The second is that treatment should principally and logically be long-term and that it be continued as long as is reasonable in each individual case, even up to old age.

The first point of view has been expressed in recent publications suggesting an increased risk of endometrial cancer in association with the use of estrogens. Procedures used in these publications, however, have been criticized by several authorities and have not fundamentally altered the opinion of adherents of the second approach and of the participants in this workshop.

Dosages

The dose of estrogen used should be the lowest effective one necessary to abolish all subjective climacteric complaints, to maintain eutrophic state of the skin and the urogenital system and to prevent osteoporosis. If for whatever reason high dosages are chosen, care should be taken to avoid hyperproliferation of the endometrium and the breasts. It can happen in practice that over-dosage occurs, because no attention was given to the level of remaining endogenous estrogen production. It is therefore of practical importance to inform the patient of the signs of estrogen over-dosage, such as pain in the breasts, cervical mucorrhoea, edema, weight gain and, of course, atypical uterine bleeding. If these symptoms occur, the estrogen dose should be reduced. In any event, an over-dose of estrogen seems less harmful when a progestagen is added for at least 10 days in the second part of the treatment cycle.

When the dosage used is adequate to deal with the symptoms, side-effects are apparently no problem.

Mode of Application and Choice of the Preparation

Oral preparations are preferred because they allow easy adjustment to the needs of the individual patient. In an intelligent, co-operative patient, oral dosages can be set according to her subjective feelings. The disadvantages of oral therapy are that gastro-intestinal symptoms occur more frequently than with other methods of administration, that patients may forget to take their tablets, or that they may take an over-dose. Some clinicians, therefore, prefer depot injections, (e.g. estradiol esters with dehydroepiandrosterone or testosterone). Others prefer long-acting implants containing estradiol, testosterone and sometimes progesterone. In these cases a regular withdrawal bleeding can be achieved if desired by intermittent administration of pro-gestagens. For the transformation of the endometrium and a complete shedding of the mucosa, progestagen therapy is required for more than 10 days. When testosterone is given to a post-menopausal patient, she should be informed of possible side-effects such as hirsutism, deepening of the voice, acne and increased libido. The combination of estrogen therapy with a progestagen in the second half of the treatment cycle may be considered more often than up to now in order to shed the proliferative endometrium periodically. Doctors and their post-menopausal patients may also have to be motivated to accept regular bleedings in this normally amenorrheic period of life.

There is a tendency to use estriol, estriol succinate, estradiol valerate and micronized estradiol (either alone or in combination with estriol) instead of preparations containing estrone. This is done apparently on the grounds that estrone has been less safe in regard to syncarcinogenicity. The evidence against estrone, however, is sus-pected to be insufficient to justify such preferences.

Estrogen administration should preferably be cyclic in order to give the target organs, the endometrium and breast, 1 week of 'rest'. The treatment schedule should imitate the normal cyclic events as much as possible. In some cases climacteric complaints might reappear during the week in which no treatment is given. Therefore it was thought reasonable to continue with low doses during this period, since even during a normal cycle estrogen production continues at a reduced level. It was however also suggested that reappearance of hot flushes during the medication-free week could serve as a useful reinforcement for the patient, reminding her how good the therapy really is for her and how badly she needs estrogens.

It still has to be shown that a regimen of 6 days on and 1 or 2 days off treatment (no medication on Saturday and Sunday) has advantages over treatment schedules that resemble more closely the normal cycle. There is also insufficient evidence to accept that continuous estriol therapy has no disadvantages.

Control of the Patient under Treatment

The patient on estrogen treatment should have a full gynaecological examination every 6 months. In addition, a vaginal smear must be taken to check the correctness of the estrogen dose used. Urine glucose and blood pressure should be monitored regularly. An examination of cholesterol, triglycerides and transaminase levels in the blood is only necessary when a special indication exists. When a non-cyclical, that is to say, unexpected, bleeding occurs, a diagnostic curettage should be performed.

Contra-indications of Estrogen Therapy

Absolute contra-indications are: severe liver disease, porphyria, cerebro-vascular diseases, deep venous thrombosis and embolism, estrogen-dependent tumours of the mammary gland, the corpus uteri or the kidney (especially when under specific therapy) and malignant melanoma. The contra-indication: thromboembolism has been copied from the pill and it has still to be shown that it applies to a low dose treatment with natural estrogens.

Relative contra-indications, which require individual decision and a more strict supervision of the patient are: estrogen-induced hypertension, cholecystitis, cholelithiasis, pancreatitis, severe cardial and nephrogenic edema and allergy to a special estrogen preparation. The indications for *dose reduction* of estrogens and for the addition of progestagens or testosterone are fibroids (myomata), endometriosis, mastopathia fibrosa cystica, over-stimulation of the endometrium, migraine and epilepsy.

In cases of hirsutism in the post-menopause an anti-androgen may be given in combination with estrogen therapy.

What are the Risks of Estrogen Therapy for the Patient?

The special risks for the older female patient are thromboembolic vascular diseases, cholecystitis–cholelithiasis and uterine carcinoma. For all these diseases predisposing factors in the family anamnesis are important. Risk factors which require extra care in the choice of preparation and dose, and therefore call for special supervision, are obesity, diabetes, hypertension, hirsutism, anovulation, long-standing cycle disturbances, sterility, nulli- or oligo-parity, heavy smoking, hyperlipaemia, immobilization and surgery.

Weighing Advantages Against Risks of Estrogen Therapy

A treatment can only be recommended when the risks of therapy are low, and in any case less than the advantages. The risks of post-menopausal estrogen replacement appear small if the general rules of therapy are followed carefully. Studies done reveal no significant rise in the incidence of thromboembolism or of endometrial and mammary carcinoma. An increase in the size of fibroids and of endometriosis can be prevented by the addition of progestagen.

On the other hand the advantages of estrogen therapy are considerable: the very unpleasant symptoms disappear; there is an increased sense of well-being, in general health, in psychic and physical fitness.

The patient's ability to work and her sex life improve in proportion to her increased self-esteem.

The beneficial influence of estrogens on the skin, the prevention of genital and breast atrophy, of hirsutism and osteoporosis are of great importance and may also partly reduce morbidity and mortality in older patients.

Conclusions

1. Estrogen replacement therapy should always be individualized according to the needs of the patient.
2. The lowest effective maintenance dose should be found for each patient.
3. A cyclical treatment is to be preferred.
4. A progestagen may be added in the second phase of the treatment cycle.
5. The patient treated with estrogens should be well-informed. She should be checked gynaecologically every six months. The frequent contact with her doctor will be of benefit to her with regard to the early detection, for example, of endometrial carcinoma. She is clearly in an advantageous position in this respect.
6. If an atypical bleeding occurs, a diagnostic curettage should be done.
7. More prospective studies on patients treated with estrogens are needed, together with basic research into indications, contra-indications, optimum dosages and effects and side-effects of estrogens. It is reassuring that such studies are being undertaken in various centres in the world.

Invited participants in the Workshop on The Estrogen Deficiency Syndrome and the Management of the Patient *were:*

I. D. Cooke (UK)   *J. W. W. Studd (UK)*
G. A. Hauser (Switzerland)   *W. H. Utian (South Africa)*
B. E. C. Nordin (UK)

10

Workshop Report

Effects and Side-effects
of Estrogen Therapy

Chairman : P. E. Lebech

Frederiksberg Hospital, Copenhagen, Denmark

Many different estrogens are used for the treatment of climacteric complaints and for the prevention of the metabolic consequences of estrogen deficiency in the post-menopause. There is an increasing body of evidence, however, that different estrogens may differ in effects and side-effects. For this reason a classification of estrogens is useful and the distinction of artificial or synthetic estrogens, such as diethylstilbestrol and ethinylestradiol, on the one hand and natural estrogens on the other may have practical importance. The natural estrogens can be divided into: 1) natural equine estrogens, containing conjugated estrogens as well as estrogens that do not occur in the human organism; and 2) natural human estrogens, genuine estrogens that occur in the normal ovulating human female, in particular estrone, estradiol-17β, estriol and conjugates of these hormones.

The expression 'ideal substitution therapy' should only be used for those therapy regimens which result in plasma concentrations of the 3 natural human estrogens comparable to those observed in the major part of the normal, ovulatory cycle. Such a therapy would lead to optimum effect with a minimum of side-effects and risks.

Data were presented indicating estradiol-17β is rapidly absorbed after oral administration: high plasma concentrations of both estrone and estradiol and their conjugates were found 15 minutes after ingestion. Conjugated estriol reached a peak 1½–2 hours later. Many of these conjugates are double conjugates. After oral administration of 2 mg estradiol and 0.5 mg estriol, the plasma level of free estradiol is at about the same level as in mid-cycle. The level of free estrone is somewhat higher and so are the levels of conjugates (Lebech)[1].

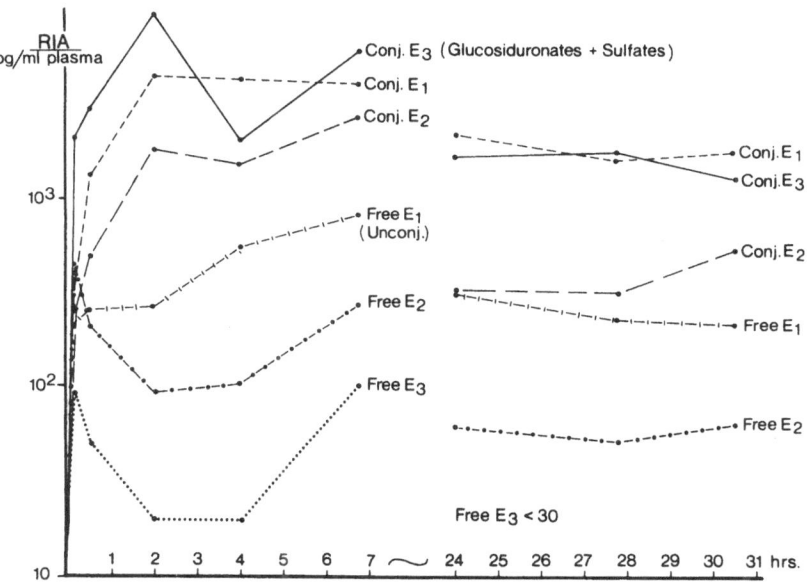

Figure 1   Oral administration of 0.56 mg 4 − [14] C-estriol S.A. 179 μCi/mg and 2 mg estradiol

All estrogens, provided they are administered in adequate dosages, can suppress the typical climacteric complaints, such as hot flushes and perspiration. The same is true of other subjective complaints of the climacteric syndrome, in as far as they are related to the typical climacteric syndrome. Higher dosages frequently are needed to obtain the state of 'well-being'. Atrophic vaginitis, urge and stress incontinence and post-menopausal skin atrophy can also be treated or prevented by estrogen therapy. The same is true for post-menopausal osteoporosis.

Such effects can be achieved with either synthetic or natural, human or equine estrogens, but on other parameters, however, effects may be qualitatively different. The effect of these 3 groups of estrogens on serum lipids may be different in the sense that natural human estrogens lower serum lipid levels, whereas synthetic estrogens may not. Åstedt and Jeppsson[2] have shown that natural estrogens do not reduce the fibrinolytic activators in the venous wall, whereas this was the case with equivalent doses of synthetic estrogen. Also no changes have been observed in thyroxine ratio and in the free thyroxine index[3].

Much emphasis has been put on the possibility of estrogen therapy without withdrawal bleeding after a period of estrogen intake. It may be necessary, however, in order to obtain all the advantages of therapy, to accept some proliferative effect on the endometrium. Therefore the best therapy is a sequential regimen in which a progestational compound is given as well on the last days of estrogen therapy. This will ensure in most cases good cycle control. Post-menopausal women on estrogen therapy, in whom such a cyclic pattern is restored, should be informed and motivated in order to improve the acceptability of this procedure.

Any irregular, unexpected bleeding under estrogen therapy needs further exploration.

As far as side-effects are concerned, natural estrogens seem to be better tolerated than synthetic. Nausea and vomiting, observed in 6–10% of women on ethinyl estradiol, is very uncommon in women using natural human estrogens (Furuhjelm and Lebech).

Mastodynia occurred in 12% of women treated with ethinyl estradiol (Rozenbaum) and about the same incidence is observed in patients on natural estrogens (Furuhjelm and Lebech). Lauritzen regarded breast tenderness as a sign of over-dose. He found that in cases of a sequential estrogen–progestagen therapy the mastodynia was sometimes worse in the progestagen phase.

Edema is a natural, physiological effect of the estrogenic hormones. Estrogens cause retention of water in the extra-cellular space. In those cases where severe water retention occurs, intermittent therapy with diuretics may be given.

Hypertension, a complication occurring occasionally in women using oral contraceptives which contain a synthetic estrogen and progestagen, is not observed as a result of therapy with natural estrogens. In post-menopausal women natural human estrogens may even have an anti-hypertensive effect (Furuhjelm and Lebech).

Hypertension as such is not an absolute contra-indication for estrogen therapy although a more careful supervision of the patient is required (Lauritzen).

Conclusion

In weighing the benefits of estrogen therapy, mental, physical and metabolic, against undesirable side-effects and risks, the conclusion has to be reached that benefits exceed the latter. This is particularly so if natural human estrogens are used, because with these estrogens the benefit/risk ratio is obviously better than with synthetic estrogens.

A sequential regimen using natural human estrogens, combined in the last days of therapy with a progestational compound, seems a promising one for the future. Further research to clarify the exact therapeutic value of the various available estrogens and treatment schedules is urgently needed.

References

1. Lebech, P. (1974). *In: The Menopause Syndrome* (R. B. Greenblatt, V. B. Mahesh and P. McDonough) pp. 199–204 (New York; Madison Press)
2. Åstedt, B. and Jeppsson, S. J. (1974). *J. Obstet. Gynaecol. Br. Commonw.*, **81**, 719
3. Kølendorf, K., Siersbaek–Nielsen, K., Hansen, J. and Friis, T. (1974). *Ugeskr. Laeg.*, **136**, 246

Invited participants in the Workshop on Effects and Side-effects of Estrogen Therapy *were*:

J. C. Burch *(USA)*
A. Comninos *(Greece)*
M. Furuhjelm *(Sweden)*
P. Kemeter *(Austria)*

Ch. Lauritzen *(West Germany)*
H. Rozenbaum *(France)*
R. Wenner *(Switzerland)*

11

Workshop Report

Estrogens and Bones

Chairman : B. E. C. Nordin

The General Infirmary, Leeds, England

Secretary: S. A. Duursma

Academisch Ziekenhuis Utrecht, Utrecht, The Netherlands

It was agreed that bone loss in women starts at or about the menopause and proceeds at about 1%/annum. In men it is slower and starts later. This loss of bone in women is associated with a steep rise in the wrist fracture rate (to about 50/10 000/annum) which does not occur in men. It was also agreed that this loss of bone is due to an increase in the rate of bone resorption rather than a fall in the rate of bone formation as Albright had originally postulated. However, there was some disagreement as to the way in which loss of estrogen causes bone resorption. Gordan thought that estrogens had an anti-catabolic effect on collagenous tissues in general and quoted reports of thin skin and reduced collagenous tissues in cases of osteoporosis. Nordin considered that bone was unduly sensitive to the action of parathyroid hormone in the absence of estrogens. Duursma thought there might be altered sensitivity of bone to growth hormone or thyroid hormone. Klotz's view was that there might be a deficiency of calcitonin. Dequeker suggested that osteoporosis was associated with growth hormone deficiency and showed increased growth hormone levels in osteo-arthrotic patients with increased bone mass.

The Effects of Estrogen and Calcium on Osteoporosis

Despite this disagreement on mechanisms, there was general agreement that estrogen therapy delayed or prevented loss of bone in post-menopausal women, and might even increase it. Furuhjelm reported a comparison of 13 post-menopausal women given 4 mg of micronized estradiol daily who were studied by X-ray densitometry and compared with 13 untreated women. The treated cases gained bone and the untreated lost bone. Dequeker reported metacarpal cortical width measurements, both retrospective and prospective, which showed significantly less bone loss in treated than untreated patients. Gordan quoted the prospective trials of Aitken and Meema which showed the same estrogen effect, and reported a reduced fracture rate in his own estrogen-treated patients. Nordin reported a prospective controlled trial in which gamma-ray absorptiometry of the forearm was used. This showed significant bone loss in the control group of 15 cases but no significant loss over 2 years in the group of 15 cases treated with ethinyl estradiol.

There was some discussion about the role of calcium in the prevention of osteoporosis. Nordin reported that his prospective trial also included a group of women treated with calcium supplements, in which no significant bone loss occurred in 2 years. He also reported that oophorectomy had little effect on bone mass in rats unless combined with a low calcium diet, when a severe loss of bone could be produced. This suggested that estrogen deficiency impaired the organ's ability to adapt to a low calcium intake. He thought that the beneficial effect of calcium supplements (and the reported effect of calcium infusions in osteoporosis) was due to parathyroid gland suppression and consequent reduced PTH-mediated bone resorption. However, Gordan considered that the effect of a calcium infusion on bone resorption was far too prolonged to be due simply to parathyroid switch-off.

In addition to the effects of estrogens and calcium, Dequeker reported that women treated for long periods with a progestagen had significantly more bone than untreated controls.

Biochemical Effects of the Menopause

Biochemical effects of the menopause were described by van Paassen and Duursma who studied pre- and post-menopausal women, the latter including treated and untreated cases. Their main finding was a rise in plasma calcium, phosphate and alkaline phosphatase after the menopause, which were to varying degrees reversible by estrogen therapy. The rise in plasma phosphate seemed to be due to increased tubular reabsorption of phosphate but there was no difference in PTH levels between the groups. Nordin also described a highly significant rise in the *mean* fasting urine hydroxyproline/creatinine and calcium/creatinine ratios in post-menopausal women which were wholly reversible with estrogen therapy. He suggested that these ratios should be measured at least twice in any given subject and that a value above the pre-menopausal range might possibly be regarded as an objective indication for estrogen therapy.

Another biochemical study was presented by Klotz who reported that the plasma calcitonin was higher in young women than in men (0.06 compared with 0.018 ng/ml) but fell to the male level in estrogen-deficient women. The level was restored to normal by estrogen therapy.

There was very little discussion about the difference between osteoporotic post-menopausal women with crush fractures and other post-menopausal women. It was agreed that such women generally had diminished trabecular bone. Dequeker thought this might date from childhood, whereas Nordin thought it was due to accelerated bone loss after the menopause, although he had not been able to find excessive resorption in the bone biopsies of these cases. He had found that osteoporotic women *as a group* tended to be more 'estrogen deficient' than other post-menopausal women due to a slightly reduced mean plasma androstenedione level, but the most striking abnormality in these patients was malabsorption of calcium. This was not due to vitamin D deficiency. It could be improved by estrogen therapy or with large doses of vitamin D (about 10–20 000 u daily); and responded completely to 1–2 μg of 1αOHD$_3$ or 1.25 (OH)$_2$D$_3$. It was probably due to suppression of renal 1-hydroxylase by the raised plasma calcium and/or plasma phosphate and/or reduced PTH levels of the estrogen-deficient state. Nordin thought that post-menopausal osteoporosis with crush fractures was due to the combination of estrogen deficiency with malabsorption of calcium, similar to the combination of oophorectomy and low calcium diet which caused such striking loss of bone in rats.

Invited participants in the Workshop on Estrogens and Bones *were:*

J. L. Ambrus (USA)	G. S. Gordan (USA)
W. Cyran (West Germany)	H.-P. Klotz (France)
J. Dequeker (Belgium)	M. Notelovitz (USA)
S. A. Duursma (The Netherlands)	H. C. van Paassen (The Netherlands)
M. Furuhjelm (Sweden)	

12

Workshop Report

Lipids and Estrogens

Chairman : U. Larsson-Cohn

Linköping University, Linköping, Sweden

Introduction

Mortality from cardio-vascular disease before the 50th year of age is many times higher among men than women. It has therefore been suggested that female ovarian hormones, e.g. estrogens, might have some protective effect against this disease. This hypothesis is still a question of debate and arguments in favour and against it are readily available. However, it has been clearly shown by the Veterans' Administration Drug Lipid Cooperative Study that long-term treatment with conjugated estrogens has no appreciable effect on the plasma cholesterol levels of men with a history of myocardial infarction.

Synthetic estrogens influence lipid metabolism in several ways. One of the more important of these is enzyme induction within the liver cell, with increased synthesis of the protein part (apoprotein) of lipoproteins as a consequence. This is most evident for the lipoprotein family called Very Low Density Lipoproteins (VLDL = pre-β lipoproteins), that transports lipids from the liver out into the circulation. As VLDL are high in triglycerides, the most obvious results will be elevated plasma concentration of that lipid fraction.

Estrogens also reduce post-heparin lipolytic activity (also called the 'clearing factor') and therefore reduce the rate with which plasma is cleared from chylomicrons or exogenously-administered triglycerides. This has been interpreted by some authors as indicating that raised triglycerides levels could be due to reduced disappearance rate from plasma. Most investigators seem to feel, however, that such a mechanism could be of only minor importance in the present context.

Another, probably more important, estrogen effect is elevation of the plasma concentration of the phospholipid-rich high density lipo-proteins (HDL = α-lipoproteins), e.g. the lipoproteins that mainly carry fats from the periphery to the liver.

As a consequence an increased part of the total plasma cholesterol will be found in this lipoprotein family. According to several reports there exists an inverse correlation between the amount of HDL in plasma and the risk of acquiring cardio-vascular disease. These alterations are therefore probably an important positive sign of the effects of estrogens on the lipid metabolism.

Natural estrogens, e.g. estrone, estradiol and estriol and also estra-diol valerianate, seem to have a less-profound influence on the metabolism of fats. This means that they do not raise the plasma concentration of triglycerides and that they may in part even have an opposite effect. From just this point of view natural estrogens are probably preferable for post-menopausal estrogen replacement therapy. On the other hand they also probably increase the HDL less than some synthetic estrogens do.

The three most common situations when women are subject to increased estrogen stimulation are worth discussing.

Pregnancy

During pregnancy the following alterations of the lipids have been reported: HDL and VLDL levels increase by 25–50%, while the elevation of the low-density lipoproteins (LDL = β-lipoproteins) is less impressive. Plasma concentrations of cholesterol and phospholipids are raised up to 50% and the levels of triglycerides usually 300–400%. These alterations are probably useful for the growing fetus. The eventual implications for the woman who went through pregnancy are not known.

Combined Oral Contraceptive Treatment

There are many reports describing the effects of combined oral contra-ceptives on various aspects of lipid metabolism. Some of these findings described are more or less in disagreement with each other, which might at least partly be due to differences in the experimental design, in the selection of the subjects taking part in the studies, in the laboratory methods that were employed and in the composition of the drugs that were studied.

Most investigators, however, have found raised levels of plasma triglycerides. In a few cases the plasma concentration of phospholipids has been determined and found to be increased. The level of cholesterol has been reported to be either moderately increased, unchanged, or moderately decreased. Post-heparin lipiolytic activity is usually reduced, but as mentioned previously, this has probably little significance in the present context.

In evaluating the literature concerning the effects of combined oral contraceptives on lipid metabolism, it is important to realize that many progestagens (gestagens) are more or less anti-estrogenic in this respect, e.g. they counteract the triglyceride-increasing influence of estrogens.

According to one or two very brief communications the short-term effects of oral contraceptives on the plasma triglyceride level may be minimized if the estrogen content is reduced from 50 μg to 30 μg per tablet, and if the gestagen has strong anti-estrogenic properties. The long-term effects of changes in lipid metabolism that may be induced by combined oral contraceptives are completely unknown.

Post-menopausal Estrogen Replacement Therapy

There are surprisingly few reports concerning the effects of estrogen administration on the lipid status of post-menopausal women. According to some recent investigations micronized estradiol-17β given orally has a tendency to reduce plasma levels of triglycerides and cholesterol. A more thorough investigation of this effect on the lipid metabolism is therefore highly warranted.

Synthetic estrogens raise plasma concentrations of triglycerides and phospholipids and seem to have a tendency to lower the cholesterol level. Although no completely comparable studies are available, estradiol valerianate and conjugated equine estrogens seem to have similar but less-marked effects. Both ethinyl estradiol and estradiol valerianate raise the HDL in plasma and also the proportion of the total plasma cholesterol that is transported within this lipoprotein family. This is probably to be looked upon as a positive consequence.

Judging from the limited data available, it would seem that post-menopausal estrogen replacement treatment does not induce changes in the plasma lipid spectrum that could be considered alarming. It may even be that the long-term effects could have a positive influence on the ageing female organism. There is, however, an urgent need for more well-controlled studies of the influence of various types of estrogens in different dose levels on post-menopausal lipid and lipoprotein metabolism.

Invited participants in the Workshop on Lipids and Estrogens *were:*

M. Furuhjelm (Sweden)   R. Punnonen (Finland)
P. Kicovic (The Netherlands)   L. Rauramo (Finland)
P. B. Lebech (Denmark)   W. H. Utian (South Africa)
W. D. Odell (USA)

13

Workshop Report

Estrogens and Clotting Factors

Chairman : J. L. Ambrus

State University of New York at Buffalo, Buffalo, New York, USA

Introduction

We are rapidly approaching a time when, in western countries, young girls will start to take oral contraceptives in their middle teens and continue on such medication throughout their reproductive lives, except for short periods when they discontinue medication in order to become pregnant. They will take estrogens in the years around their menopause and throughout their post-menopausal years. Thus they will live the majority of their lives under increased estrogenic influence. All this time many will be concerned about possible thromboembolic complications, despite the fact that the incidence of thromboembolism, even under these conditions, is very low.

There is no doubt that the use of oral contraceptives is associated with a definite, albeit only slightly increased risk of such complications, and there is also no doubt that steroid hormones can influence blood levels of components of blood coagulation and fibrinolytic systems. Data to confirm the latter aspect were presented at this workshop by Ambrus, Notelovitz, Davies and Poller. As far as oral contraceptives are concerned, such changes are clearly due to the estrogenic component of these products and not to the progestational component. Progestagens, used alone, do not alter the blood coagulation system (Ambrus).

There are indications that different estrogens may have different effects and that natural estrogens in particular are less likely to induce such changes than are synthetic estrogens such as ethinyl estradiol. This may have implications for estrogen therapy in the years around the menopause and in the post-menopause, because in these phases of life it is mainly natural estrogens that are used. The following evidence for such differences between natural and synthetic estrogens was presented:

1. Ambrus and Notelovitz reached the same conclusions concerning the effect of estrogens on anti-thrombin III levels, although they studied somewhat different clinical groups and used different laboratory methods:

   a) There is no difference in anti-thrombin III levels between normal males and females.
   b) In pregnant women at term a profound fall in anti-thrombin III blood level was observed.
   c) Oral contraceptives containing synthetic estrogens produced a fall in these levels, but less than that induced by pregnancy.
   d) In post-menopausal women the use of conjugated natural estrogens produced a fall which was less than that induced by oral contraceptives. In fact the values found did not differ significantly from those observed in untreated controls.

2. Davies presented data suggesting that therapy with ethinyl estradiol resulted in greater and more wide-spread changes in the levels of blood coagulation factors (VII, IX and X) than did the natural estrogen, estriol-succinate.

Assessment of Risk

When estrogens do induce changes in the levels of various components of the blood coagulation and fibrinolysis systems—natural estrogens having this quality to a lesser extent than synthetic estrogens—the question remains as to the significance of such changes in regard to the risk of thromboembolism. Data were presented which indicate that appropriate pre-treatment screening may result in detection of those women who are particularly at risk of developing thrombo-embolic complications. A group of about 350 women, comprising those on oral contraceptives and controls using other, non-hormonal methods of contraception, was studied for about 6000 cycles over about 2 years, to reveal only four cases of possible thromboembolic complications. One of these was in the control group, the others in the group of women using oral contraceptives. However, all these four women had abnormal blood coagulation patterns before they entered the study, abnormal patterns which continued to deteriorate as time progressed (Ambrus).

It has also been reported that plasminogen levels increased under estrogen therapy (Davies, Ambrus). This may represent increased activity of the fibrinolytic system, to balance changes that are induced in the coagulation system. When these systems do not balance each other, thromboembolism can occasionally result. The increase in plasminogen levels may, however, also be interpreted as a lack of activation of plasminogen to plasmin. This would then lead to de-creased activity of the fibrinolytic system (Ambrus). Davies, on the other hand, found that in those cases where plasminogen levels were increased under ethinyl estradiol therapy euglobulin lysis activity was increased as well, indicating an increased activity of the fibrinolytic system (Davies).

The changes in the coagulation system induced by therapy with estrogens, obviously do not progress continuously and do not therefore result in extremely high levels. The changes level off, usually after 3–9 months of therapy. Occasionally the changes regress between the 9th and 24th month of treatment (Ambrus).

The effect of estrogens on platelet function are rather complex. Essentially the rate at which the platelets aggregated in response to collagen and adrenalin was accelerated after estriolsuccinate therapy, and the platelet stickiness (adhesion) was reduced. The relevance of these *in vitro* findings is conjectural and other workers using various estrogens have reported variable findings with platelet function tests (Davies).

Some results presented indicate that it may be possible to develop oral contraceptives, acceptable both from the gynaecological point of view and with regard to efficacy, which do not influence blood coagulation. Low dose estrogen (alternate day) and progestagen therapy with two regimens were found to produce no effect on blood coagulation, platelet function and fibrinolysis (Ambrus).

Conclusions

Estrogen therapy, even during the post-menopause, should aim at the lowest possible effective dose level. This, and appropriate pre-treatment haematological screening to eliminate the patient at risk (who can then be treated otherwise), might well remove the risk of thrombo-embolism and the fear thereof.

Invited participants in the Workshop on Estrogens and Clotting Factors *were:*

J. A. Davies *(UK)*

M. E. Gahwyler *(USA)*

G. S. Gordan *(USA)*

T. Ikeda *(Japan)*

M. Notelovitz *(USA)*

D. D. Oram *(UK)*

L. Poller *(UK)*

L. Tax *(The Netherlands)*

A. Thénot *(France)*

E. Vázquez *(Mexico)*

14

Workshop Report

Estrogens and Endometrial Cancer

Chairman : R. B. Greenblatt

Medical College of Georgia, Augusta, Georgia, USA

Secretary: R. D. Gambrell, Jr.

Wilford Hall USAF Medical Center, Lackland, Texas, USA

Discussion about a possible association between estrogens and endometrial and breast cancer is almost as old as estrogen therapy itself. Certainly there have been arguments which seem to point to a causal relationship, the result of pharmacological studies and some clinical observations. But there have been many, if not more, data indicating that no such relationship exists.

The difficulties in confirming or denying a causal relationship between the intake of any chemical substance and cancer are considerable. The case of the possible carcinogenicity of estrogen used in the post-menopause is no different.

Recent publications have presented new evidence alleging such a connection[1-3]. Participants took advantage of this session to review the difficulties mentioned above, using some of the recent publications as examples of where the pitfalls are and how they can lead to the wrong conclusions.

Regrettably the authors of these publications, although invited, were unable to attend this congress session. D. C. Smith initially accepted the invitation to be on the programme but had to withdraw at the very last moment.

Histological Bias

The histological bias in the diagnosis of endometrial cancer is considerable. It is often the case that pseudo-malignancy, atypical
hyperplasia, adenomatous hyperplasia and cancer *in situ* are recorded
in a conscious or subconscious effort to effect an early and ready cure.
Any clinician of long experience can quote cases showing how often
histological bias favours malignancy, thus altering the true incidence
of endometrial carcinoma.

Skilled pathologists often differ in the interpretation of histological
findings and may even disagree on the significance of the same histological section.

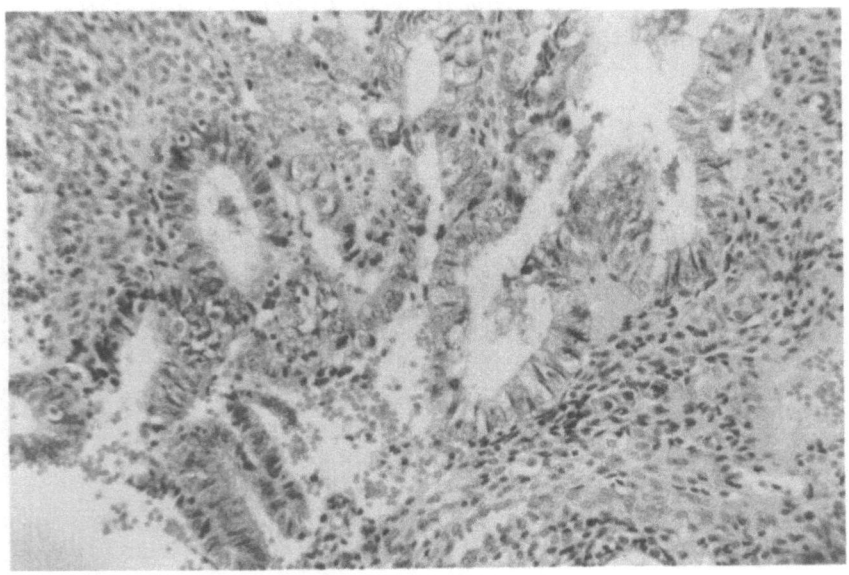

Figure 1 Diagnosis of endometrial carcinoma made by one pathologist, and
carcinoma *in situ* by the consulting pathologist

The following example may illustrate this. The histological picture
of Figure 1 was diagnosed as advanced endometrial cancer by one
pathologist and as carcinoma *in situ* by another.

The patient was treated with several courses of an oral progestagen. The endometrium changed and became functional and secretory (Figure 2).

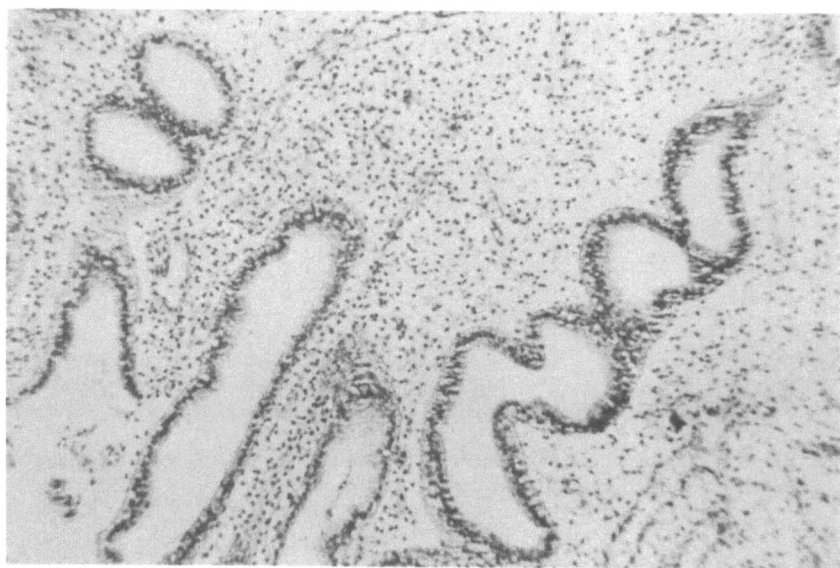

Figure 2 Same patient: Note complete change to a secretory endometrium following a 10-day course of an oral progestagen

Fifteen years later, during which two full-term pregnancies occurred, the uterus was removed. No evidence of atypia or malignancy was found. The administration of a progestagen during 10–15 days may indeed be a differential diagnostic measure in those cases where diagnosis is doubtful. If a complete secretory change results, the diagnosis is not carcinoma. Illustrations of this are given in Figures 3 and 4. If such changes do not occur, the diagnosis of carcinoma is sustained and proper measures should be taken.

Estrogen therapy often induces abnormal bleeding in a woman with a latent endometrial cancer. A diagnostic curettage, which would be the normal procedure under the circumstances, would in all probability uncover the silent cancer before invasion occurred. This sequence may be regarded as an unexpected benefit for women for

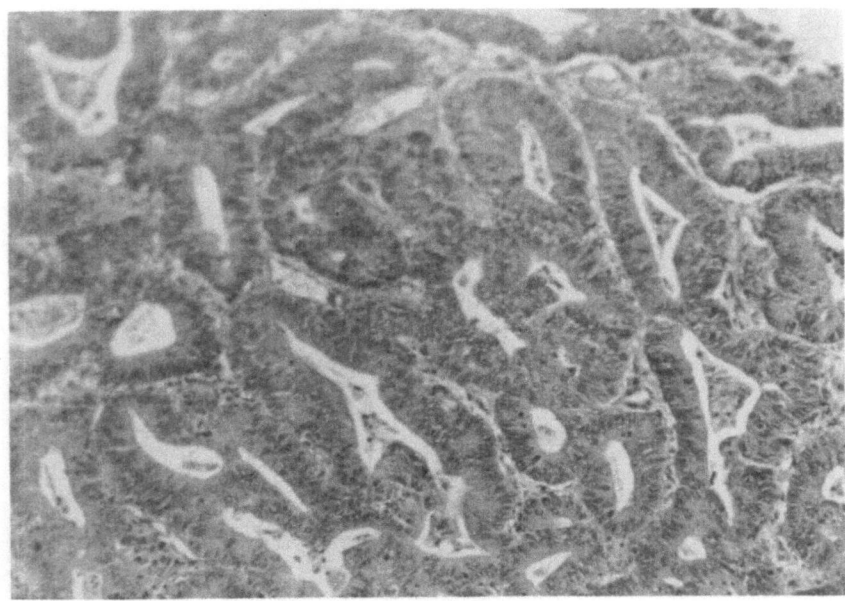

Figure 3 Diagnoses ranged from adenomatous hyperplasia, and cancer *in situ* to well-differentiated endometrial cancer

whom a later diagnosis of cancer could mean a life of despair, or even prove fatal. Figures 5 and 6 illustrate this.

Morbidity and Mortality Statistics

According to the National Cancer Survey endometrial cancer in the US has increased two-fold: from 10.3 to 20/100 000 from 1947 to

Table 1 Cancer incidence and mortality in USA—white population. Note great reduction in mortality from endometrial cancer. (From the National Cancer Survey–1969–71)

	Incidence/100 000		Death rate/100 000	
	1947	1969–71	1950	1970
Breast	72.6	72	24.2	25.2
Corpus uteri	10.3	20	9.1	4

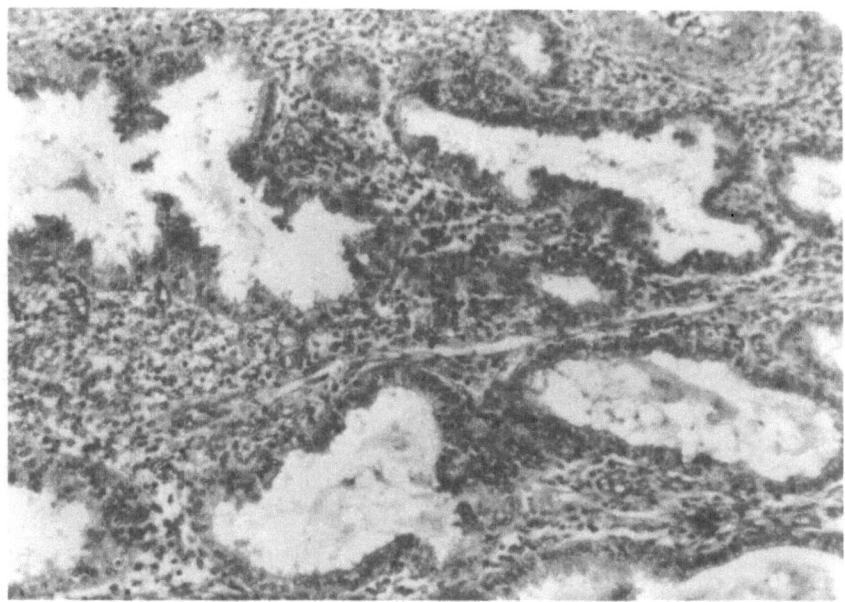

Figure 4 Same patient: Note complete change to a secretory endometrium following a 10-day course of an oral progestagen

1969–71. The mortality rate, however, has decreased from 9.1 to 4/100 000 in the same period.

These findings are not easy to explain. Certainly management of endometrial cancer has not changed over the past three decades. Perhaps earlier diagnosis and bias toward malignancy has permitted a greater chance of survival. The 1976 report of the American Cancer Society states that 'Increases in corpus cancer incidence in older women have recently been reported. Also an enhanced risk has been linked to a growing use of exogenous estrogens. The data (provided in table form) predate these reports and do not suggest any increase in incidence, in part because of fewer intact uteri at risk due to increase in hysterectomy not for cancer'. One might conclude that estrogen use is associated with an increased chance of hysterectomy, rather than an increased chance of dying from endometrial cancer (Greenblatt).

In the state of Connecticut, there appears to have been an increased diagnosis of endometrial carcinoma over the past 20 years. Table 2

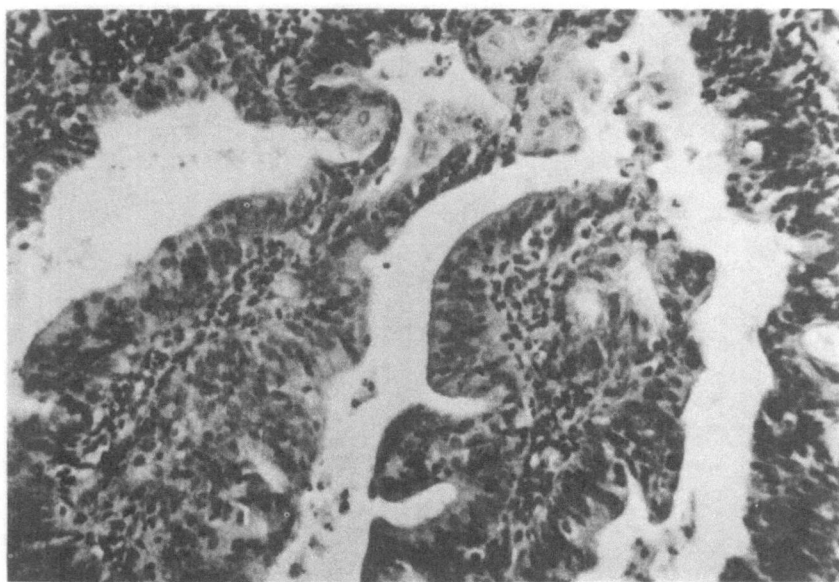

Figure 5 Papillary adenocarcinoma of the endometrium in a 53-year-old with mild uterine bleeding of several weeks duration that started after 3 months of sequential estrogen–progestagen therapy

presents the reported number of diagnoses of uterine corpus cancer, principally endometrial carcinoma.

Table 2 Increasing diagnosis of cancer of uterine corpus. (Connecticut Tumor Registry—Connecticut State Department of Health)

	Year of diagnosis							
	1953		1963		1968		1973	
Age (years)	*No*	*Rate**	*No*	*Rate*	*No*	*Rate*	*No*	*Rate*
All ages	134	(12.1)	270	(19.6)	310	(20.5)	457	(28.5)
40–49	15	(10.1)	46	(24.8)	35	(18.0)	68	(35.7)
50–59	43	(35.2)	67	(46.2)	94	(56.2)	151	(83.4)
60–69	39	(43.2)	92	(83.5)	103	(86.9)	129	(97.0)
70–79	23	(46.0)	44	(64.9)	58	(75.3)	75	(89.5)

Provided by J. T. Flannery, Director, CSTR; Casey, M. J. and Davids, R. S.
* Rate/100 000 female population.

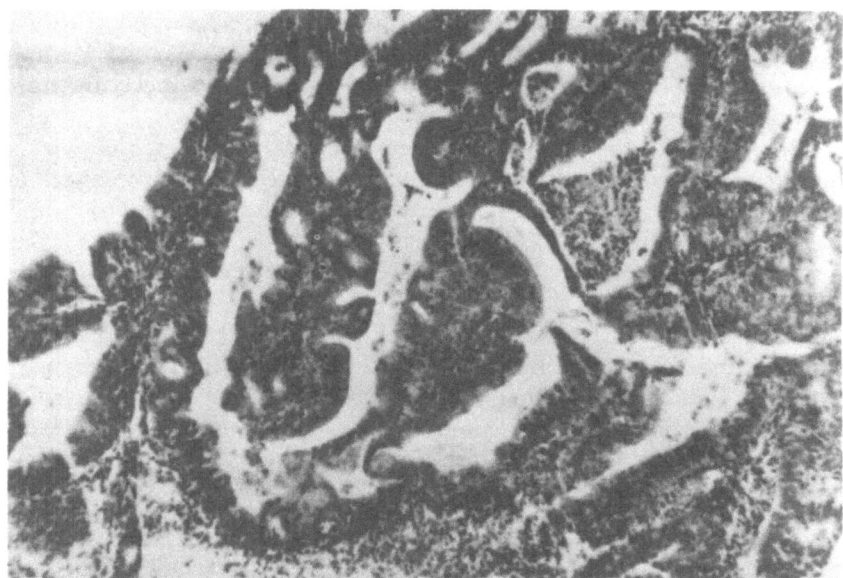

Figure 6 Same patient: No change in endometrial pathology occurred from a 10-day course of an oral progestagen. It must be assumed that a silent neoplasia was present before start of therapy. Hormone therapy contributed to an early diagnosis and an ultimate beneficial result

The trend toward increased diagnosis of cancer of the uterine corpus is obvious. It is significant at the level $p < 0.001$ for all ages except the 70–79 year age group, where the significance level is $p < 0.01$ when

Table 3 Decreasing incidence of invasive cancer of uterine cervix. (Connecticut Tumor Registry—Connecticut State Department of Health)

	Year of diagnosis							
	1953		1963		1968		1973	
Age (years)	No	Rate*	No	Rate	No	Rate	No	Rate
All ages	244	(22.1)	161	(11.7)	182	(12.0)	180	(11.2)
40–49	57	(38.2)	48	(25.8)	41	(21.0)	37	(19.4)
50–59	69	(56.2)	40	(27.6)	51	(30.5)	46	(25.4)
60–69	46	(50.9)	27	(24.5)	27	(22.8)	22	(16.5)
70–79	10	(20.0)	15	(22.1)	21	(27.3)	32	(38.2)

Provided by J. T. Flannery, Director, CSTR; Casey, M. J. and Davids, R. S.
* Rate/100 000 female population.

Chi-squared analysis, using the Yates correction, was applied to the rates reported for 1953 and 1973. (Casey, M. J., Davids, R. and Flannery, J. T. unpublished analysis data from the Connecticut State Tumor Registry 1976.)

The increased diagnosis of endometrial cancer has coincided with a significant ($p < 0.001$) decrease in the incidence of invasive cancer of the uterine cervix reported in the 20-year period between 1953 and 1973. This is shown in Table 3.

Increased vigilance by both physicians and patients may contribute to the changing patterns (Casey).

However, Cramer and co-workers of the National Cancer Institute, in updating information from the Third National Cancer Survey and from the Connecticut Registry, found *no* increase in the incidence of endometrial cancer in the United States[4]. They pointed out, in fact, that correcting the figures for 'unspecified' cancer of the uterus indicates that the incidence of endometrial cancer is actually declining.

Bias due to Retrospective Studies

The three recent publications, based on retrospective data, conclude that estrogen therapy increases the risk of endometrial carcinoma. In one study, conducted in Los Angeles and reported by Ziel and Finkle[2], the pair-matching of the comparison subjects was by age, postal zip code of residence and length of membership in the Kaiser Foundation Health Plans. In the second study, conducted in Seattle and reported by Smith *et al.*[1], matching consisted of age and year of diagnosis among women in the same hospital who were treated for cervical, ovarian or vulval cancer. A search of the medical records of women with endometrial cancer indicated that they were 4.5–7.6 more likely to have received estrogen therapy than their pair-matched compeers.

A third study having bearing on this issue was described by Mack *et al.*[3]. They reported that in a retirement community near Los Angeles, patients with endometrial cancer were 8.0 times more likely to have received endogenous estrogen than their compeers without this condition.

The 'cases' were matched with women selected to be within one year of age, to have the same marital status and to have arrived at the retirement home within six months of their pair-matched partners. More compeers than patients were alive at the time of the study.

In the three studies cited, at least five variables—singly or in combination—could have been significant, but not causal, factors in the observed association between exogenous estrogens and endometrial cancer:

1. Possible use of estrogens for peri-menopausal bleeding caused by pre-existing endometrial carcinoma.
2. Greater frequency of diagnostic examinations (dilation and curettage, aspiration, biopsy or jet washes) among the women taking estrogens.
3. Possible misinterpretation of estrogen-induced hyperplasia as neoplasia.
4. Socio-economic differences and other disproportions between comparison groups.
5. Eligibility bias in selection of comparison groups.

If the cancers in the reported studies were indeed diagnosed because of earlier examination or more frequent screening, staging should show them to be early cancers. Amplifying data presented by D. C. Smith at the FDA committee meeting on Dec. 16, 1975,

Table 4 Note that 95.5% of the endometrial cancer reported by D. C. Smith were in stage 0–1 and that deep invasion was found in only 1% in the estrogen-treated in comparison to 18% in the non-treated group. (Reproduced from John Studd. *Br. Med. J.*, 8 May 1976, *p.* 1144)

Stage	Estrogen group	Non-estrogen group
0 (hyperplasia)	16	7
1	129	115
2	6	20
3	2	15
4	0	7
Total	153	164
Invasive	17%	44%
Deeply invasive	1%	18%

indicated that estrogen-treated women did indeed have earlier tumours. The figures would then reflect early detection and cure, not cause and effect (Table 4, presented by Studd).

With respect to eligibility bias in the selection of subjects for comparison, consideration must be given to the question of whether the cases and comparison groups in all three studies were representative.

In the Los Angeles study, for example, only those cases of endometrial carcinoma that were reported to the tumour registry were included. The authors stated that there was uncertainty about completeness of reporting, particularly before 1971. Yet the cases were selected from the tumour registry in the last half of 1970. It is likely that omission of unreported cases caused ascertainment bias, because women receiving estrogen therapy were probably seen more often by their physician and were therefore more likely to have their cancers diagnosed and reported to the registry.

Dunn and Bradbury[5] studied patients with untreated endometrial carcinoma or post-menopausal vaginal bleeding who were admitted to their service in Iowa City and given complete evaluations. These investigators properly controlled the study for the most important factor; why the patient came to their attention in the first place. They also took into account age, weight, parity, history of abortion, use of contraceptive measures, menstrual history, presence or absence of hypertension or diabetes mellitus, age at menopause and socio-economic status. There were 139 women in the final series, all of them medically indigent, who had been admitted because of vaginal bleeding. Uterine curettage was performed in each of these patients. Only obesity and infertility were found to correlate with endometrial cancer. Of those found to have endometrial carcinoma, 28.6% had received estrogen therapy. Among the non-cancer group, the figure was 27.5%, a trivial, statistically insignificant difference. This negative finding unfortunately was not mentioned in the discussion on estrogens and endometrial carcinoma appearing in the February–March 1976 FDA *Drug Bulletin* (Gordan).

Retrospective studies do have inherent pitfalls. One of them is associated with the choice of controls. In one study[1], socio-economic status was disregarded. The estrogen-treated subjects were of high socio-economic level, while controls were from a much lower economic category. Patients treated with estrogen, over-represented in the higher socio-economic levels, are followed more closely and have D and C more readily for any kind of abnormal bleeding or spotting. Hence detection is more frequent (Lauritzen).

Clinical Observations

Clinical experience, however useful, cannot be regarded as hard evidence to accept or refute an association between estrogen therapy and cancer. It is reassuring that a number of participating clinicians with long-standing experience with estrogen therapy expressed their considered opinion that the risk, if it is increased, is still extremely remote. Some attach great value in this respect to: 1) either cyclical administration, 2) the combination of estrogen therapy with progestagens, or 3) to the use of specific estrogens such as estriol and estradiol. No unanimity on these three points was reached, although the first and second found much approval.

Prospective Studies

The final answer to the question as to whether estrogens may be associated with an increased risk of endometrial cancer will only be given when the results of prospective studies are known. Only prospective studies can avoid the methodological pitfalls described above. It is appreciated that the organization of such studies is not easy, but this is no reason to neglect them.

Conclusions

The recent studies alleging an increased risk of endometrial carcinoma in women under estrogen therapy are open to serious criticism. The consensus of participants appears to support the view that there is no direct etiological relationship between endometrial cancer in women and estrogen therapy. In view of the inherent defects of retrospective studies, the urgent need for prospective investigations was emphasized. Close supervision of these women and adequate action when abnormal bleeding occurs is necessary. Under these conditions the benefits to be derived from estrogen therapy far outweigh the risks in general and the putative risk of endometrial carcinoma in particular.

References

1. Smith, D. C., Prentice, R. and Thompson, D. J. (1975). Association of exogenous estrogen and endometrial carcinoma. *N. Engl. J. Med.*, **293**, 1164
2. Ziel, H. K. and Finkle, W. D. (1975). Increased risk of endometrial carcinoma among users of conjugated estrogens. *N. Engl. J. Med.*, **293**, 1167

3. Mack, T. M., Pike, M. C., Henderson, B. E., Pfeffer, R. I., Gerkins, V. R., Arthur, M. and Brown, S. E. (1976). Estrogens and endometrial cancer in a retirement community. *N. Engl. J. Med.*, **294**, 1262
4. Cramer, D. W., Cutler, S. J. and Christine, B. (1974). Trends in the incidence of endometrial cancer in the United States. *Gynecol. Oncol.*, **2**, 130
5. Dunn, L. J. and Bradbury, J. T. (1967). Endocrine factors in endometrial carcinoma: a preliminary report. *Am. J. Obstet. Gynecol.*, **97**, 465

Invited participants in the Workshop on Estrogens and Endometrial Cancer were:

M. Albeaux-Fernet (France)
J. C. Burch (USA)
M. J. Casey (USA)
G. S. Gordan (USA)
D. Kaskarelis (Greece)
P. Kemeter (Austria)

Ch. Lauritzen (West Germany)
E. Nishida (Japan)
A. Onnis (Italy)
L. Rauramo (Finland)
E. Schleyer-Saunders (UK)
J. W. W. Studd (UK)

Section B

Selected Papers Presented at the
Congress

15

Cross-cultural Factors that Affect Age of Menopause

Marcha Flint

Montclair State College, Upper Montclair, New Jersey, USA

Studies of factors that affect the age of menopause are nowhere nearly as clearly defined as are those factors thought to influence the age of menarche. Moreover, menopausal age, specifically, and how it is affected by specific factors have been studied by few researchers, although there have been many references to the believed effects of these factors on delayed or early menopause. In this paper I will review some aspects of reproductive history, genetic factors, pathological, geographical and socio-economic factors, and a secular trend as they may influence age of menopause cross-culturally.

REPRODUCTIVE HISTORY

Age of Menarche

One of the most constant beliefs alluded to from the early 1900s to the 1970s is that an early age of menarche indicates a late age at menopause[1-3]. With the exception of Sanes'[4] 1916 study in the United States and that of Wood's[5] in Australia in 1971 this correlation has been generally unproven. This is true for Denmark[6], Great Britain[7], The Netherlands[8], South Africa[9] and the United States[10].

Further, one can question both Sanes' and Wood's findings. Sanes[4] said that both an abnormally early (12 years or less) or abnormally late (18 years or more) age at menarche tended to favour an early menopause. Wood's[5] study, on the other hand, considered an early menarcheal age as 13 years old and this is not considered to be early by most researchers[9, 11]. One investigator's work has contradicted both Sanes' and Wood's findings. Stopes[12] found that patients who had a late menarcheal age (over 16 years) also had a late menopause.

Of course, these studies that asked women for their ages at menarche and menopause generally employed the retrospective method of eliciting information. While this methodology may be valid[13] for specific populations where these reproductive landmarks have important significance and would, therefore, need to be known, questions about accuracy of recall ability should be noted for most studies. Frommer[14] has cautioned that women tend to 'round off' these dates at 5-year intervals in recalling age of menopause, at 45 or 50 years rather than noting those years in between these dates. Ideally, to test the correlation of menarcheal age to menopausal age accurately, a prospective study using a probit or logit analysis would be best.

Realistically, there are also a great many problems in trying to correlate these two ages. The factors that may affect each woman's reproductive history from menarche to menopause are myriad. Numbers of miscarriages, diet, infectious diseases, general health, and psychological stress are just a few of these. In 35 years of reproductive life, there may be just too many factors intervening that must be considered, in trying to correlate age of menarche with age of menopause.

Parity

Another aspect of reproductive history that has been accepted as affecting menopausal age is parity. As early as 1897, Currier[15] stated that a series of childbirths which rapidly succeeded each other, and continuous lactation exhausted the reproductive forces and was a forerunner of an early menopause. Sanes[16] was one of the first to refute this belief and showed in an analysis of 621 cases, that the larger the number of pregnancies the later the onset of the menopause. Several other researchers have supported Sanes' findings in various countries: Australia (Wood[5]); Italy (Principe and Delaurentiis[17]); Mexico (Soberon, Colderon and Goldzieher[18]); South Africa (Benjamin[9]);

and the United States (Norris[19]). But others refute any correlation between parity and age at menopause[6-8, 10, 20].

A few authors have tried to correlate multiparous and nulliparous women with age of menopause, as well. They found that women who have had no children reached an age of menopause sooner than those with children[5, 9, 17, 19]. Two allied studies of this factor were those of Jaszmann, van Lith and Zaat[8] in The Netherlands and Hauser *et al.* in Israel[21] which found that unmarried women had an earlier menopause age than married women. Both these studies also equated a gravidity of nil with this unmarried group. MacMahon and Worcester[10], however, found no significant difference in age of menopause between unmarried and married women.

Two other studies have also correlated parity and socio-economic class with menopause age. One of these was done by McKinlay, Jeffries and Thompson[11] in England and the other was that of Soberon, Colderon and Goldzieher[18] in Mexico. McKinlay's group separated their female subjects by age into either low (manual) or high (non-manual) socio-economic status based on their husband's occupations. They concluded that parity appeared to delay the menopause only for younger (age 45–49) women of higher socio-economic status rather than older women (age 50–54)[11]. Soberon's team[18] studied 222 low income clinic patients and 1262 more affluent private patients in relation to parity and menopausal age. A group of post-menopausal nuns from a convent in Mexico City were included as part of this latter sample.

This Mexican study showed that the clinic group exhibited no correlation between high parity and late menopause, while the private patients did show this correlation[18]. There are several aspects of this second study that may be questioned. The sample groups were primarily Catholic and there would, therefore, have been little contraceptive use, but there may have been abortions performed although these were not recorded. What effects this may have had on parity rates is unknown. Also, there is the possibility of a skewed analysis due to the small number of clinic patients as compared to private patients, and finally, the group of nuns comprised most of the unmarried nulliparous women included in the private patient group. This inclusion might well have biased this sample.

One final aspect of parity has been studied only by Pumpianski[20] in Israel. This is the effect of numbers of abortions on age of menopause. He found that the greater were the number of abortions, the earlier was the onset of menopause. This subject is one that should be given more study, particularly with the increases of legal abortion cross-culturally today.

The Pill

Since the Pill has only been widely used for about 15 years, we do not as yet know its effect on age of natural menopause. McCary noted that 'the age at menopause is not dependent upon the maturation and discharge of all eggs contained in the ovaries' . . . 'The use of the Pill (which prevents ovulation) may in some instances cover up the onset of menopause, but there is no evidence that it will delay it[22]. The recent work of Costoff and Mahesh[23] also shows that the menopause is not a result of a depletion of all primordial follicles in the ageing ovary.

A control study of the effect of the Pill on early or late natural menopausal age is about due as women who were in their thirties in the 1960s would be coming into menopausal age now.

GENETIC FACTORS

Race

Unlike aspects of reproductive history which may or may not be correlated with age of menopause, race is generally agreed to affect this age. In the 1920s Kisch[2] flatly stated that race did affect age of menopause, and in the 1930s Stopes supported this belief by noting that 'Northern and Anglo-Saxon types tend to be older in years when it arrives than women of Southern or oriental races'[12].

Later studies by Abramson et al.[24] among South African Zulu women and by Benjamin[9] among South African white women further support Kisch's[2] statement. Abramson et al.[24] found the age of menopause among their subjects to have a mean of 49.2 years while Benjamin's yielded a mean of 48.7 years[9]. A more recent study by Frere[25] of South African Bantu and white women gave a probit mean menopausal age of 50.7 years for Bantus and 51.44 years for whites which he felt to be significant. In the United States, MacMahon and Worcester[10] compared 169 black and 1219 white women's ages at natural menopause and found the differences in their mean ages, 49.21 and 50.02 years, respectively, not to be significant.

The discrepancy of an earlier menopausal age for South African white women studied by Benjamin[9], as compared to a later menopausal age for white women elsewhere when they were compared with non-white women, can possibly be explained. Abramson et al.'s[24] study of South African women only numbered 33 subjects compared to 1000 studied by Benjamin[9]. The South African Zulu mean menopausal age, therefore, would not necessarily be as representative of a true mean as the larger South African white sample.

By the same token, the unequal sample size of blacks compared to whites in MacMahon and Worcester's[10] United States study might well have skewed their similar mean age findings.

Familial Patterns

A few authors have suggested that heredity may have a relationship to age of menopause, but there are no twin, sister or mother–daughter studies to prove this belief as there have been with age of menarche (Bolk[26]; Damon et al.[13]; Gould and Gould[27]; Petri[28]; Popenhoe[29]; and Young, Zoli and Gallagher[30]).

Currier was one of the first writers to note a familial pattern in menopausal age. 'Lateness of menopause is characteristic in some families'[15]. McCary also stated that 'The age at which the menopause occurs appears to be related, like the menarche, to an inborn genetic factor and to general health'[22]. Way too said 'Our work suggests that the menopausal age is predetermined genetically'[31].

Way's[31] findings, however, are based on mothers and daughters who had had operative menopauses because of hysterectomies due to carcinoma of the body of the uterus. The familial menopause brought on by this operation is certainly not natural and cannot be considered as genetic, but this does not exclude the possibility that carcinoma of the uterus body may not be genetically timed to be expressed in both mothers and daughters around a specific age. More work needs to be undertaken of kinship effects on menopause age, preferably with longitudinal studies between generations, and in different cultures.

PATHOLOGICAL FACTORS

Diseases

There have been few studies of specific diseases that affect age of menopause. One of the earliest noted was obesity and both Currier[15] and Stopes[12] felt that it accelerated menopausal age. Sanes[16] also found eight cases of obesity associated with early menopause as were nine patients with syphilis; he also stated that 15 patients with a cardio-vascular disease, five with gout and ten with diabetes had a late menopause. Unfortunately these sample sizes are too small to be statistically significant.

Several other investigators have associated specific diseases with either early or late menopause. Those diseases associated with an early age are pruritus senilis, cancer of the ovaries, cancer of the vulva and hernia[32]. Those diseases associated with a late age include: cancer of the body of the uterus[9, 31-33]; cancer of the breast[32, 34]; cancer of the cervix[9]; diabetes[9, 31, 33, 35]; fibroids[32]; and polyps[31].

In Great Britain, both Awon[33] and Way[31] stated that there was also an association between cancer of the uterus and diabetes as well as their individual association with late age of menopause. Only Way postulated that 'Overactivity of the anterior pituitary may lead to many different manifestations such as fibroids, diabetes or cancer of the uterus and these could have happened singly or in combination, and part of this complex may have been a retarded menopause'[31]. This theory should be investigated further.

GEOGRAPHICAL FACTORS

Climate

Menopause age and its effect by climate has not been studied since the 1930s and there is little conclusive evidence for any correlation of these factors, even before this date.

Currier stated that women living in tropical climate have their menopause at 30 to 40 years while in temperate climate it is at 45 to 60 years[15]. This was refuted by Leuf[3] and Kisch[2] who noted that those living in climates which were tropical had late menopausal ages. Only Curjel wrote that 'Climate and other accidental factors are not con-sidered to exert the same influence on the cessation of the reproductive functions as on its commencement'[36].

Altitude

Another geographical factor, altitude, and its effect on menopausal age has only been studied by Flint[37] and Cruz-Coke[38]. Flint found that at 2283 m, the mean menopause age for Indian women of the Rajput caste was 47.3 years as compared with these same women who lived at 300 m and had a mean menopause age of 48.9 years—a 1.5 year difference[37]. Cruz-Coke also found an acceleration of over one year in age of menopause in Chilean women living over 3000 m when compared to those living below 1000 m[38]. The reason for this difference between low altitude and higher altitude women's ages at menopause is not known. It is felt, however, by Flint and Cruz-Coke that the lowered oxygen pressure at the higher altitudes may have something to do with this[37, 38], much as it has to do with a later age of menarche noted by Frisancho and Baker[39] in comparing high to low altitude Quechua females.

SOCIO-ECONOMIC FACTORS

One factor that has been consistently associated with menopausal age is socio-economic level. It is believed that women in the upper socio-economic classes achieve their menopause later than those in the lower classes. Kisch[2] noted that German working women achieved their menopause earlier than those in the upper classes, but McKinlay, Jeffries and Thompson[11] in England compared socio-economic status based on husband's occupation (without a relationship to parity) with earlier or later menopause age and found no significant differences of age between lower and higher occupational groups. MacMahon and Worcester[10] also found no correlation between family income and menopausal age.

Jaszmann, van Lith and Zaat[8] considered education as a factor that might affect menopause age but found no correlation here. Urban versus rural habitats also showed no correlations with menopause age[6, 10].

Too little research has been done on socio-economic factors and their effects on menopause age to flatly state that there are no correlations. Certainly socio-economic conditions affect one's level of nutrition, education and health. The higher one's socio-economic status, the more likely it would be that one's nutrition, health and education levels would be bettered. These factors might well mitigate physiological and psychological stresses and possibly slow down the ageing process which would delay the age of menopause.

SECULAR TREND

It is believed that menopausal age is being achieved later; however, this is an extremely difficult idea to prove or disprove. A century ago women didn't live beyond 48 years of age in the United States[40], and in other cultures, for example, India and parts of Africa, women seldom lived beyond their fortieth year. Today with an increase in the life expectancy of women we may well be able to study a secular trend, if one is present, for later menopausal age with longitudinal cross-cultural studies. Backman[41], analysing European data, first suggested that menopause began at 40 in ancient times, was 45 in the period 1500 to 1830 A.D. and in 1948 was 48. Thus menopause would appear to have been delayed about 3 years in the last hundred years in Europe. Frommer[14] in 1964 found the mean age of menopause in Great Britain to be 50.2 years, an increase of 4 years since the mid-19th century, and MacMahon and Worcester[10] reported a median age of 49.7 years in the United States in 1960–62, 1.8 years later than Norris'[19] mean age of menopause in this century.

Other authors, however, do not believe that the age of menopause has changed at any time. Burch and Gunz[42] reported an average age of 50 years for New Zealand women in 1967 and noted that older studies of these women also reported a modal age of 50 years. McKinlay, Jeffries and Thompson in 1972 reported a median menopause of 50.78 years for London women and stated that 'There is no conclusive evidence of an increase in the age of menopause over the last century'[11].

To refute Backman's findings, in 1970 Amundsen and Diers[43] reported that while the Classical period first recorded 40 years as the typical age for menopause, later an age of 50 years was given with a range of from 35 to 60 years. Post also concluded from his search of medieval writings that 'The menopause figures especially are so wide ranging as to invite wholesale rejection' ... 'It seems possible to hypothesize for the periods to which these sources relate, an age at menopause no dissimilar to those apparent in mid-twentieth century'[44].

Even MacMahon and Worcester, who cited earlier ages of menopause in the United States than their own, stated that any differences in age at menopause in the last 50 years could have been due to methodological problems[10]. One of these is the lack of homogenous methodology for all researchers. Most have used the retrospective method of eliciting menopause age, while others have used probit analyses or logit analyses. Each of these methods gives different ages, using the same data.

Other problems in secular trend research involve lack of continuity of menopausal ages over more than a limited number of years for some countries, small sample sizes of under 500 women, and a frequent difficulty in getting accurate mean menopause age because most cross-cultural literature records the age of menopause at from 45 to 50 years and does not give a specific mean age. These same problems may be said to affect the study of menopause age correlated with any of the various factors previously discussed, as well.

SUMMARY

The aspects of reproductive history that seem to affect menopausal age are parity and marriage versus non-marriage and abortion. Genetic factors like race and familial patterns have been generally accepted also as affecting this age. Diseases such as diabetes, fibroids, polyps and cancers of the body of the uterus, cervix and breast are associated with late age of menopause while cancers of the ovaries and vulva, pruritus senilis and hernia are associated with early menopausal age. The only geographical factor known so far that affects menopausal age is altitude and it has been found to accelerate this age.

No socio-economic factors have been conclusively correlated to this age. The question of whether or not there is a secular trend for a later age at menopause has not been shown, as yet.

Taking all these factors together, there are very few that do affect menopause age, and there is a real need for more research to be undertaken cross culturally of those factors that might affect the age at which menopause is achieved.

References

1. Kelly, G. L. (1961). Menopause. In A. Ellis and A. Abarbanel (eds.) *Encyclopedia of Sexual Behavior*. 718 (New York: Hawthorn Books)
2. Kisch, H. (1928). *The Sexual Life of Women and the Physiological and Hygienic Aspects* (translated by M. Eden Paul). (New York: Allied Book Company)
3. Leuf, A. H. F. (1902). *Gynecology, Obstetrics, Menopause*. (Philadelphia: The Medical Council)

4. Sanes, K. I. (1916). Menstrual statistics—Study based on 4500 menstrual histories. *Am. J. Obstet. Dis. Women Child.*, **73**, 93

5. Wood, E. C. (1971). The Female Reproductive System. In J. Krupinski and A. Stoller (eds.) *The Health of the Metropolis: The Findings of the Melbourne Health and Social Survey.* 52 (Sidney: Halstead Press)

6. Clausager-Madsen, L. and Ytting, H. (1942). Undersogelserouer menarchensog menopausens indtraeden i byog landbefolkningen. *Nord. Med.*, **16**(3), 677

7. Council of the Medical Women's Federation. (1933). An Investigation of the Menopause in One Thousand Women. *Lancet*, **i**, 106

8. Jaszmann, L., van Lith, N. O. and Zaat, J. C. A. (1969). The age at menopause in the Netherlands—The statistical analysis of a survey. *Int. J.Fertil.*, **14**, 106

9. Benjamin, F. (1960). The age of the menarche and of the menopause in white South African women and certain factors influencing these times. *S. Afr. Med. J.*, **34**, 316

10. MacMahon, B. and Worcester, J. (1966). *Age at Menopause, United States—1960–62* in U.S. Dept. of Health, Education and Welfare, Public Health Service, National Center for Health Statistics, Series 11, Number 19. (Washington, D.C.: U.S. Government Printing Office)

11. McKinlay, S., Jeffries, M. and Thompson, B. (1972). An investigation of age at menopause. *J. Biosocial Sci.*, **4**, 161

12. Stopes, M. C. (1936). *Changes of Life in Men and Women.* (London: Putnam Publishers)

13. Damon, A., Damon, S., Reed, R. and Valadian, I. (1969). Age at menarche of mothers and daughters with a note on accuracy of recall. *Hum. Biol.*, **41**(2), 161

14. Frommer, D. J. (1964). Changing age of the menopause. *Br. Med. J.*, **2**, 349

15. Currier, A. (1897). *The Menopause*, p. 1897. (New York: D. Appleton and Co.)

16. Sanes, K. I. (1918). The Age of Menopause: A Statistical Study, Translations of the Section on Obstetrics, Gynecology and Abdominal Surgery of the American Medical Association, 258

17. Principe, S. and Delaurentiis, G. (1958). Esiste una correlazione tra eta al menarca ed eta alla menopause. *Riv. Ostet. Ginecol.*, **13**(11), 673

18. Soberon, J., Colderon, J. and Goldzieher, J. (1966). Relation of parity to age at menopause. *Am. J. Obstet. Gynecol.*, **96**, 96

19. Norris, C. C. (1919). The menopause. *Am. J. Obstet. Dis. Women Child.*, **79**, 767

20. Pumpianski, R. (1967). Age at natural menopause. *Harefuah*, **77**, 513

21. Hauser, G. A., Remen, U., Valaer, M., Erb, H., Muller, T. and Obiri, J. (1963). Menarche and menopause in Israel. *Gynaecologia*, **155**, 38

22. McCary, J. (1973). *Sexual Myths and Fallacies.* (New York: Van Nostrand Reinhold Co.)

23. Costoff, A. and Mahesh, V. (1975). Primordial follicles with normal oocytes in the ovaries of postmenopausal women. *J. Am. Geriatr. Soc.*, **23**(5), 93

24. Abramson, J. H., Gampel, B., Slome, C. and Scotch, N. (1960). Age at menopause of urban Zulu women. *Science*, **132**, 356

25. Frere, G. (1971). Mean age at menopause and menarche in South Africa. *S. Afr. J. Med. Sci*, **36**, 21

26. Bolk, L. (1923). The menarche in Dutch women and its precipitated appearance in the younger generation. *K. Akad. Wet. Amsterdam*, **26**(2), 650

27. Gould, H. and Gould, M. (1932). Age of first menstruation in mothers and daughters. *J. Am. Med. Ass.*, **98**(16), 1349

28. Petri, E. (1934). Untersuchungen zur Erbbedingtheit der Menarche. *Z. Morphol. Anthropol.*, **23**, 43

29. Popenhoe, P. (1928). Inheritance of age of onset of menstruation. *Eugen. News*, **13**(7), 101

30. Young, H. B., Zoli, A. and Gallagher, J. R. (1963). Events of puberty in 111 Florence girls. *Am. J. Dis. Child.*, **106**, 568

31. Way, S. (1954). The aetiology of carcinoma of the body of the uterus. *J. Obstet. Gynaecol. Br. Emp.*, **61**, 46

32. Hauser, G. A., Müller, T., Valaer, M., Erb, H., Obiri, J. A., Remen, U. and Vanaanen, P. (1961). Der Zusammenhang zweichen gynäkologischen Krankheiten und dem Menopausealter. *Gynaecologia*, **152**, 270

33. Awon, M. P. (1959). Association between climacteria haemorrhage, carcinoma of the body of the uterus and diabetes mellitus. *J. Obstet. Gynaecol. Br. Emp.*, **64**, 50

34. Hems, G. (1974). The menopause and breast cancer. *Lancet*, **1**, 362

35. Arduino, F. and de Cruz Ferreira, F. (1958). A menarche e a menopausa na mulher diabetica e pre-diabetica. *Arq. Bras. Endocrinol. Metabol.*, **7**(1), 77

36. Curjel, D. (1920). The reproductive life of Indian women. *Indian J. Med. Res.*, **8**(2), 366

37. Flint, Marcha. (1974). Altitude Effect on Age of Menopause. Paper presented at the *American Anthropological Association's 73rd Annual Convention*, Mexico City, November, 1974

38. Cruz-Coke, R. (1967). Genetic Characteristics of High Altitude in Chile. Paper presented at the *Meeting of Investigators on Population Biology of Altitude*, Washington, D.C., November 13–17

39. Frisancho, R. and Baker, P. (1970). Altitude and growth: a study of the patterns of physical growth of a high altitude Peruvian Quechua population. *Am. J. Phys. Anthropol.* **32**(2), 279

40. Gifford-Jones, W. (1969). *On Being a Woman: The Modern Women's Guide to Gynecology*. (New York: The MacMillan Co.)

41. Backman, von Gaston. (1948). Die beschleunigte Entwicklung der Jugend, verfrühte Menarche, verspätete Menopause, verlängerte Lebensdauer. *Acta Anat.*, **4**, 421

42. Burch, P. R. and Gunz, F. W. (1967). The distribution of the menopausal age in New Zealand: an exploratory study. *N.Z. Med. J.*, **66**, 6

43. Admundsen, D. W. and Diers, C. J. (1969). The age of menopause in classical Greece and Rome. *Hum. Biol.*, **41**, 125

44. Post, J. B. (1971). Ages at menarche and menopause: some medieval authorities. *Popul. Stud. (London)*, **25**, 43

16

The Influence of Estrogens on the Psyche in Climacteric and Post-menopausal Women

Mirjam Furuhjelm and P. Fedor-Freybergh

Sabbatsberg Hospital, Karolinska Institutet, Stockholm, Sweden

Hormonal factors are known to have an influence on psychological function in human beings. The climacteric and the post-menopause are consequences of the declining production of hormones from the ovaries. In the reproductive feedback system a gap develops, where there is no suppression of LRH and gonadotropic hormones, and large amounts of FSH and LH are secreted into the blood stream. The serum levels of FSH and LH in post-menopausal women exceed those found during the fertile life by a factor of 30 or more. This change in the hormonal status influences many functions of the body. Many psychological symptoms developing during this period of life are probably dependant upon the hormonal changes. However, between the ages of 50 and 60 many other changes take place in the life of the woman. The children have grown up and are leaving home; the woman feels that she is no longer young and beautiful, difficulties on her place at work may appear, she may be replaced by younger people, her husband is no longer progressing in his career, and so on.

It is difficult to determine to what extent the psychological changes which take place are dependant on the hormonal situation and to what degree they arise from other changes in the woman's life. The course of the climacteric is thus dependant on many different factors. The ovarian deficiency causes a disturbance in the hormonal balance on the hypothalamic–diencephalic level, latent symptoms emerge and the compensatory mechanism of the personality gives way.

Many climacteric and post-menopausal women complain about different psychological symptoms: nervousness, irritability, sleep difficulties, depression, impaired memory and decreasing libido. Jaszmann[1] found a considerable incidence of fatigue and depression in a study of Dutch women in the post-menopause. Kopera[2] has described a decrease in energy and a greater tendency toward nervous exhaustion among climacteric women. Krüskemper[3] studied 59 women between the ages of 40 and 50 with the Minnesota Multiphasic Personality Inventory (MMPI). The climacteric women involved in his study had no signs of somatic diseases but showed all the fears and limitations usually seen in patients with psychological disorders. They showed a higher rate of hypocondria, depression and anxiety than a control group of women in the fertile age.

Many attempts have previously been made to treat post-menopausal women suffering from psycho-pathological symptoms with estrogens. Already in the 1920s Biel reported good results after treatment with estrogens for depression, irritability and sleep disturbances. Hawkinson[4] treated 1000 patients with menopausal symptoms including depression with estrogens and found a significant improvement. The same experience was noted by several other authors. Bowman and Bender[5]; Werner[6] and others. In Sweden Ingvarsson[7] treated 28 women suffering from menopausal psychosis with estradiol; 71% of them improved significantly. Dorothea Kerr[8] treated depressed menopausal women either with hormones, psychotropic drugs or psychotherapy and found that the hormonal treatment was superior to the others.

Schildtkraut[9] claimed that a central adrenergic dysfunction is the biochemical base for the development of a depression. The gonadal hormones have an influence on the central adrenergic function by their regulatory effect upon the monoaminoxidase activity. Klaiber[10] found that the plasma MAO activity in women with estrogen deficiency was higher than in normally menstruating women. With estrogen treatment the MAO activity returned to levels found in the preovulatory phase of the menstrual cycle.

It is difficult to draw any conclusions about the effect of hormonal treatment on the mental function of a person without using reliable objective psychological tests. Rauramo et al.[11] used psychological tests to determine the psychological changes of women who had undergone oophorectomy. They found that castrated women without estrogen substitution were more irritable and tearful than the control group.

OWN INVESTIGATIONS

At the Sabbatsberg hospital we have tested climacteric and post-menopausal women with different psychological tests before and after treatment with estrogen for 1, 3 and 6 months in order to clarify the influence of estrogens upon their mental function.

The following psychodiagnostic test methods were adopted for the study: Hamilton depression rating scale, Sabbatsberg depression self-rating scale and Sabbatsberg sexual self-rating scale (Fedor-Freybergh and Dornic[12]), Sabbatsberg psychosomatic rating scale (to be published), colour word test, konzentration Verlaufs test (KVT), auditory perception test, choice reaction time, perception prove test, attention test (Fedor-Freybergh et al.[13]). Before the experiment a personality inventory test according to Eysenck was undertaken.

Material

The material consisted of:

Group I.—27 climacteric women, mean age 46.4 years. They had irregular menstruation amd similar psychosomatic symptoms, namely hot flushes, nervousness, anxiety, depression, sleep disturbances, etc. which symptoms had developed recently and from which they had not suffered before. They were treated with 1 mg estradiol valerate (Progynon) a day for 12 days followed by 1 mg estradiol valerate and 30 µg L-norgestrel for 10 days, followed by 0.5 mg estradiol valerate for 6 days.

Group II.—26 post-menopausal women, mean age 54.6 years who had been amenorrheic for at least 12 months, and who had the same psychosomatic symptoms as Group I. They were treated with 2 mg of estradiol valerate for 12 days followed by 2 mg estradiol valerate and 30 µg L-norgestrel for 10 days, followed by 1 mg estradiol valerate for 6 days.

Group III.—25 post-menopausal women, mean age 54.0 years, 12 of whom were given placebo tablets and 13 were treated with 2 mg estradiol valerate for 3 months. The patients were tested before and after treatment.

RESULTS

Hormonal Determinations

The climacteric women in Group I had normal values of FSH and LH and serum levels of low polar estrogens (LPE; estradiol-17β + estrone) corresponding to values found during the middle of the proliferative phase of the menstrual cycle. The post-menopausal women had elevated values of FSH and LH and very low values of LPE in the blood serum (Figure 1).

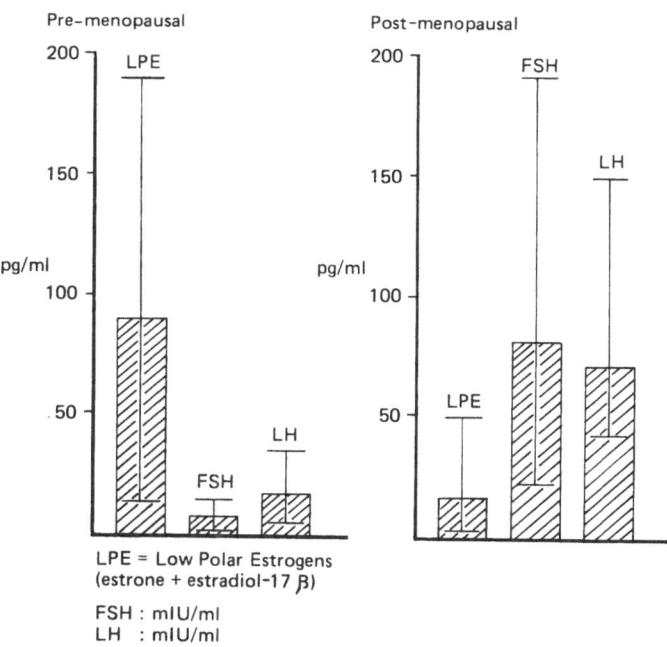

Figure 1   Hormone levels in Group I and II pre- and post-menopausal women

General and Gynaecological Examination

All women underwent a general and a gynaecological examination before the treatment started. In addition, the following blood tests were oarried out: Haemoglobin, MCHC, serum iron, cholesterol, blood lipids, proteins and transaminases GOT and GPT. No significant changes to these values occurred during the treatment. When estradiol valerate 1 mg was administered, the levels of estrogens in the blood increased by 50 pg/ml to a level corresponding to values normally found during the follicular phase of the menstrual cycle. At the 2 mg dose, the blood serum estrogen values increased by 100 pg/ml.

Results of Psychological Tests

(1) It appears from the EPI test that all groups had a higher grade of neuroticism in comparison with a standard population (Figure 2).

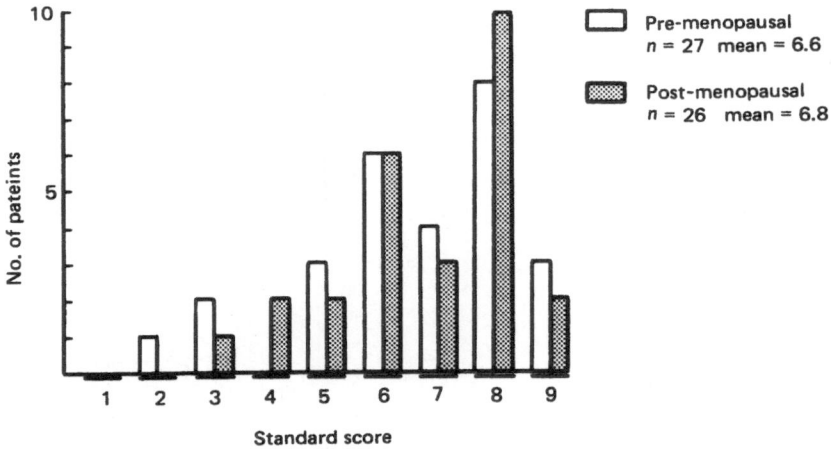

Figure 2   Neuroticism tested by the Eysenck Personality Inventory

(2) All the three groups had a tendency toward depressive symptons. With the Hamilton rating scale for depression and the Sabbatsberg depression self-rating scale (SDSRS) a significant improvement was observed even after 1 month of treatment and was more pronounced after 3 and especially after 6 months of treatment. There was a strong correlation between the two tests (Figure 3).

(3) Performance tests were used for estimation of the choice reaction time (Figure 4), attention (Figure 5), short-term memory (Figure 6) and concentration (Figure 7). The estrogen treatment improved

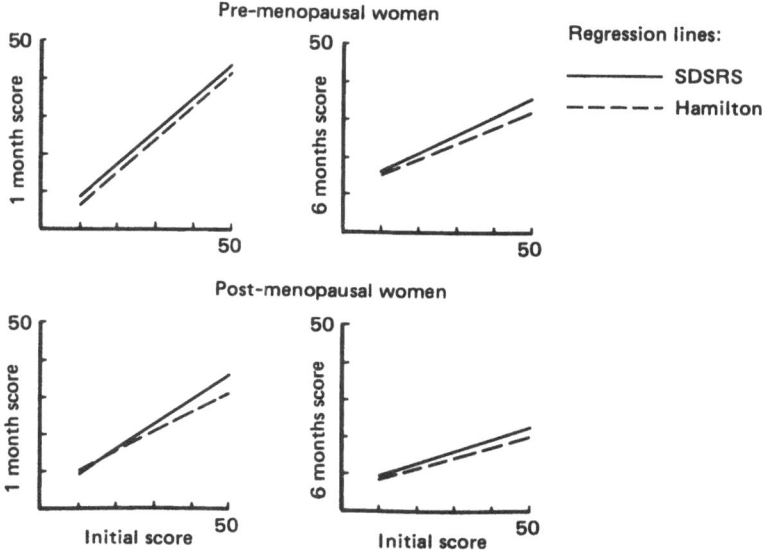

Figure 3 Comparison between Hamilton Rating Scale for depression and Sabbatsberg Depression Self-Rating Scale (SDSRS)

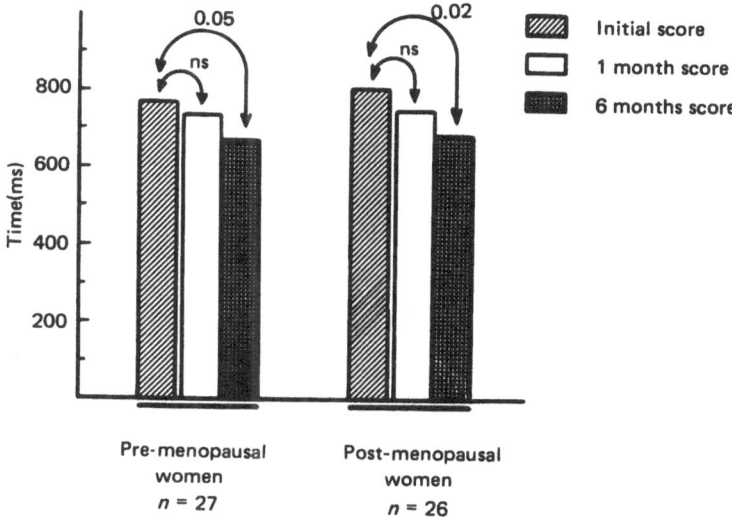

Figure 4 Choice reaction time

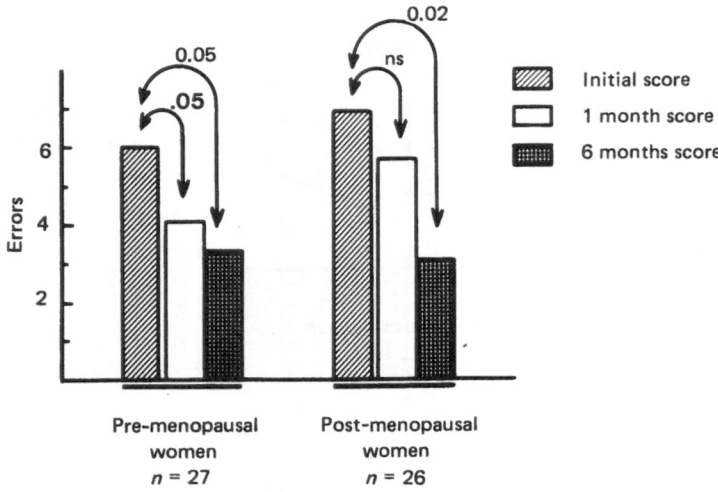

Figure 5 U-test (for estimation of attention)

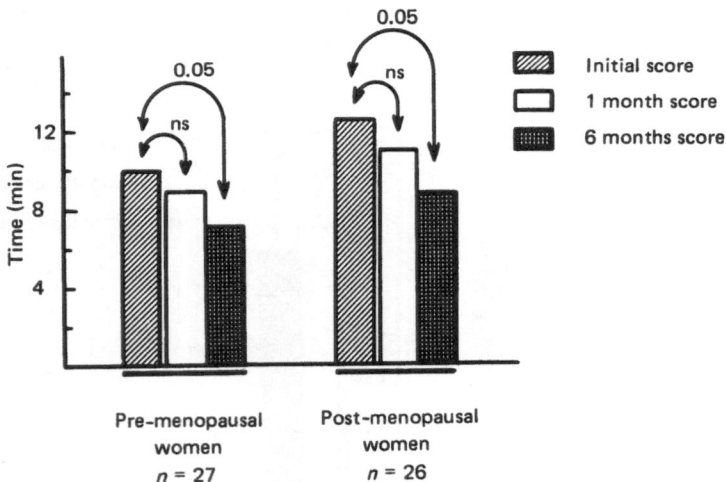

Figure 6 Visual search test (for short-term memory)

mental performance in all these tests. They revealed a tendency to stop the decline in the perceptive and cognitive skills as well as in concentration ability and memory. The more complicated tasks showed a greater improvement than the more simple ones.

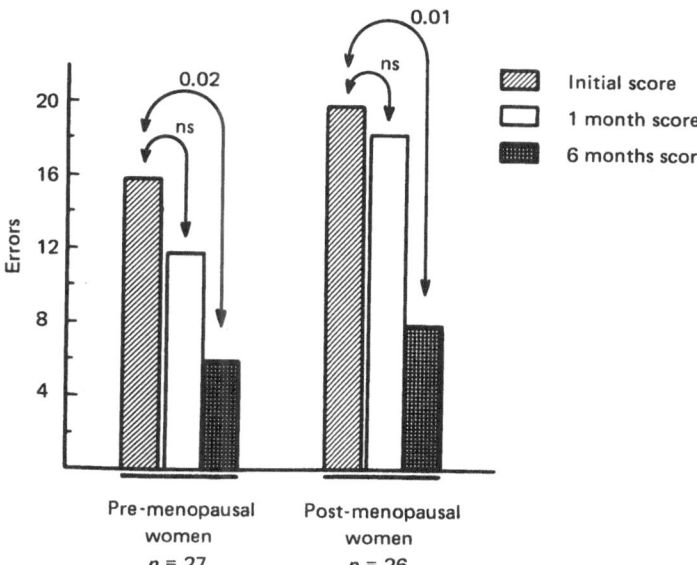

Figure 7 KVT test (for estimation of concentration)

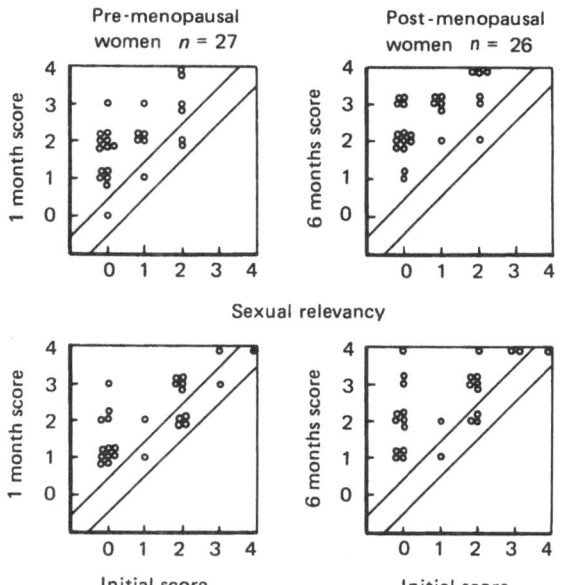

Figure 8 Sabbatsberg sexual rating scale

(4) Sexuality was estimated by using the Sabbatsberg sexual rating scale. The patients answered questions regarding libido, experience of sexual activity, orgasm, sexual fantasy and sexual relevancy (Figure 8). The estrogen medication resulted in a greater libido, greater experience of pleasure and greater satisfaction. The patients who initially had low values had the best improvement and this was most pronounced after 6 months of treatment.

(5) Psychosomatic disorders with emphasis on the mental symptoms, i.e. anxiety, restlessness, uneasiness, etc. showed a clear improvement (Figure 9).

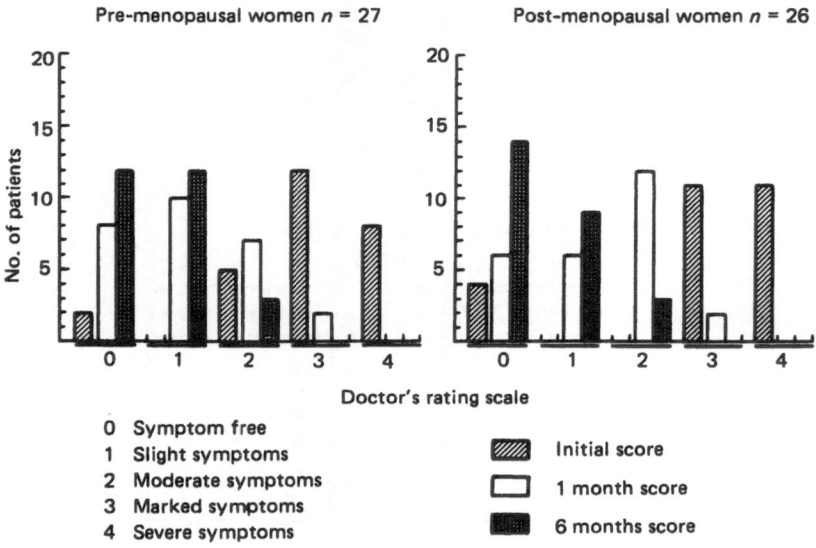

Figure 9   Sabbatsberg psychosomatic rating scale

In all tests there was a significant difference between the patients on placebo who did not improve at all and the estrogen-treated groups.

CONCLUSIONS

An estrogen treatment which is started immediately after the menopause or when patients start to complain about climacteric symptoms is of great importance from a preventive point of view. By treatment with estrogens it is possible to avoid deterioration of mental performance and to avoid the development of depression. It is also possible to reverse changes which have already appeared.

References

1. Jaszmann, L. (1973). Epidemiology of climacteric and post-climacteric complaints. *Ageing and Estrogens. Front. Horm. Res.*, **2**, 22 (Karger, Basel)
2. Kopera, H. (1973). Estrogens and psychic functions. *Ageing and Estrogens. Front. Horm. Res.*, **2**, 118
3. Krüskemper, G. (1975). Results of psychological testing (MMPI) in climacteric women. *Estrogens in the Post-Menopause. Front. Horm. Res.*, **3**, 105
4. Hawkinson, L. F. (1938). The menopausal syndrome. *J. Am. Med. Soc.*, **111**, 390
5. Bowman, K. M. and Bender, L. (1932). *Am. J. Psychiatr.*, **11**, 867
6. Werner, A. A. (1936). *Acta Neurol. Belg.*, **35**, 1076
7. Ingvarsson, G. (1971). Hormone treated cases of menopausal psychosis. *Acta Psychiatr. Scand.*, **26**, 2
8. Kerr, M. D. (1968). Psychohormonal approach to the menopause. *Mod. Treat.*, **53**, 587
9. Schildkraut, J. J. (1965). The catecholamine hypothesis of affective disorders. *Am. J. Psychiatr.*, **122**, 509
10. Klaiber, E. (1974). *First World Congress of Biological Psychiatry*. Buenos Aires
11. Rauramo, L., Lagerspetz, K., Engblom, P. and Punnonen, R. (1975). The effect of castration and peroral estrogen therapy on some psychological functions. *Estrogens in the Post-Menopause. Front. Horm. Res.*, **3**, 94
12. Fedor-Freybergh, P. and Dornic, S. (1975). Performance on some attention and memory tasks as a function of hormonal therapy. Reports from the Institute of applied psychology. The University of Stockholm No. 68
13. Fedor-Freybergh, P., Hjelmqvist, M. and Zador, G. (1976). Psychodiagnostic follow-up of Neovletta—a new low-dose oral contraceptive. *Acta Obstet. Gynecol. Scand.* (in press)

17

A Double-Blind Study into the Influence of Estriol on a Number of Psychological Tests in Post-menopausal Women

G. Vanhulle
University of Louvain (KUL), Louvain, Belgium and

R. Demol
University of Ghent, Ghent, Belgium

The aim of the present study was to investigate the influence of estrogen therapy on some psychological functions in post-menopausal women. Twenty-six subjects, all volunteers, were divided into placebo and experimental groups and examined before and after 3 months of estrogen or placebo treatment.

Each subject was tested on the following parameters: subjective estimation of the health state; visual and auditive memory; concentration; learning ability; reaction time and alertness; tempo of work and attention. The experiment revealed differences between subjects receiving estrogens and those receiving placebos in relation to attention, alertness and subjective estimation of their state of health. The clearest improvements were obtained in attention.

Introduction

It is generally believed that the feeling of impaired memory and the reduced powers of concentration belongs to subjective symptoms in menopausal women. A study of the literature gives rise to the hypothesis that there is decreased alertness as well as nervous exhaustion, fluctuation in mood, fatigue and diminished energy (Kopera[1], Rauramo[2], Krüskemper[3]).

The question underlying this study is 'Can these effects be corrected by estrogen administration?' A psychological experiment was done, using objective, standardized and reliable tests, to evaluate the influence of estrogen treatment, in this case with estriol, on a number of psychic functions. For this pilot study the following 6 parameters were selected: subjective estimation of the health state; visual and auditory memory; concentration; learning ability; reaction time and alertness; tempo of work and attention.

Methods

a) The Experimental Group

The study was begun with 29 volunteers, all of them nuns living in a religious community. They were selected because of their relative isolation from outside society, their regular life pattern and their participation in the experiment *as a group*. Three dropped out; two women in the placebo group as a result of nervousness, dizziness and general discomfort and one woman in the estriol group because of lack of motivation. The final sample was divided into two groups: (1) the experimental or estrogen group ($n = 11$) with an average age of 56.6 years and (2), the placebo group ($n = 15$), with an average age of 58.7 years.

The criteria for inclusion of the volunteers were:

1. That they should have had their menopause or castration at least 2 years earlier.
2. That they had no other somatic troubles except those related to their menopause.
3. That they received no hormonal treatment in the previous year.
4. And that no tranquillizers were taken in the three months prior to the study.

b) Experimental Design and Measured Parameters

This was a double-blind study: the subjects were randomly divided into two groups: one on estrogen, the other on a placebo. Neither the subjects nor the psychologist, nor any other person closely associated with the subjects, were informed as to who was getting which medication. The period of treatment was 3 months. The experimental group received 4 mg of estriol/day.

Before the medication was started, each subject was tested on all 6 parameters.

c) Psychological Tests

The following tests were carried out:

1. *Subjective estimation of the health state* was measured by the VOEG (Vragenlijst Over de Ervaren Gezondheidstoestand). The test consists of 56 statements and each statement is to be marked as 'yes' or 'no'. The test yields two scores:

   a) the 'yes-score' is the total of 'yes' answers on questions where one should expect 'no' answers (e.g. 'are you often nervous?')
   b) the 'no-score': is the total of 'no' answers on questions where one should expect 'yes' answers (e.g. 'have you been feeling well lately?')

   In the final calculations we also made a choice of 18 items regarding menopausal complaints.

2. *Memory*

   a) *Visual:* The Benton Visual Retention test was used, in which respondents have to reproduce a number of pictures.
   b) *Auditory:* The sub-test Series of Numbers of the WAIS (Wechsler Adult Intelligence Scale) was used. Respondents have to reproduce series of numbers that have been read to them.

3. *Concentration.* Two tests were used:

   a)—the substitution sub-test of the WAIS and;
   b)—the sub-test of arithmetical calculations of the GIT (Groninger Intelligence Test) where the subjects have to do a number of sums in a short time.

4. *Learning Ability* was measured by the Manual Labyrinth of Rey. In this test there are 4 boards with 9 buttons, one of which is fixed to the board. The other buttons are loose. The respondents have to find the fixed ones by trial and error and to remember where they are on the board. The score is based on the number of tries needed to find the four fixed buttons.

5. *Reaction Time and Vigilance (alertness).* We used the Wiener Reaktionsgerät of Dr. Shuhfried. Reaction time was measured in

hundredths of seconds with three sorts of programme: single visual stimuli, combined auditive and visual stimuli and multiple visual stimuli. Vigilance was measured by the number of unnecessary reactions and by the number of non-reactions.

6. *Tempo of Work and Attention* were measured by the Spot Pattern Test of Bourdon-Wiersma. In this test the respondents are instructed to mark those groups which contain 4 dots in lines of dotted patterns consisting of either 3, 4 or 5 dots. The number of lines completed is the measure of the tempo of work. The number of lines done divided by the number of mistakes made is the measure of attention.

Results

For the statistical analysis of the results of all tests we used one-sided *t*-tests since the direction was pre-determined, namely an improvement. We made the following analysis: Pre-test and post-test results from both groups were evaluated. The differences between the pre-tests and post-tests were compared statistically and an analysis of variances was made.

a) Pre-Test Results in Both Groups
The differences according to the *t*-test applied were not significant, which showed that the groups were similar in their pre-test situation.

b) Post-Test Results in Both Groups
The mean score in the estrogen-treated group was significantly better from the placebo mean score for the 'attention' parameter (at the 3% threshold level).

c) Differences of the Means of Both Groups (post-tests minus pre-tests)
For the 'subjective estimation of the health state', the results were not significant for the total 'yes'-score. For the total 'no'-score the differences were significant at the 7% threshold level. For the 18 items related to the menopause, the estrogen-treated group had better results than the placebo group on eleven items. For 3 of these items the difference was significantly better. The estrogen group mentioned pressure on the thorax less often (0.08), indicated that they suffered

perspiration less frequently when it was not warm (0.07) and were less tired in the morning (0.04).

There were no significant differences for the 'visual and auditive memory', 'concentration' and 'learning ability' parameters.

Differences in results in reaction time were not significant. The results for the 'alertness' parameter are shown in Table 1. There is only one significant difference, namely in the number of times the subjects failed to respond when single visual stimuli were given.

Table 1. Results for the parameter 'alertness'

Alertness	Programmes		
	Single visual stimuli	Combined auditive + visual	Multiple visual stimuli
Mistakes of excess	NS	NS	NS
Mistakes of omission	0.03	NS	NS

No significant differences in the results were found for tempo of work. The experimental group showed significantly better results (at the 3% threshold level) than the control group for the 'attention' parameter.

d) Analysis of Variance

After eliminating the influence of age, we found that the effect of treatment was significant on two parameters: attention (0.08) and alertness (0.07).

Discussion

The clearest results were obtained in attention. The differences between the estrogen and the placebo groups were significant in the post-test. In the analysis of variance, after eliminating the effect of age, this improvement stays significantly better. Finally by studying the differences we may conclude that the women taking estrogen had higher scores than those of the women taking the placebo. We are now examining in which aspects of attention those improvements occur.

Jaszmann[4] has shown that there are important psycho-social differences between women with regard to climacteric complaints.

Our study group is certainly biased in that its members have never been married and have never been pregnant. They also differ in education from women in the outside world. It is presumed therefore that if this study were repeated in a lay study-group, the differences would be more marked.

References

1. Kopera, H. (1973). Estrogens and psychic functions. *Front. Horm. Res.*, **2**, 118
2. Rauramo, L., Legerspetz, K., Engblom, P. and Punnonen, R. (1975). The effect of castration and peroral estrogen therapy on some psychological functions. *Front. Horm. Res.*, **3**, 94
3. Krüskemper, G. (1975). Results of psychological testing (MMPI) in climacteric women. *Front. Hormone Res.*, **3**, 105
4. Jaszmann, L. (1973). Epidemiology of climacteric and post-climacteric complaints. *Front. Horm. Res.*, **2**, 22

18

The Relation Between Androstenedione and Estrone Levels in Peri- and Post-menopausal Women

D. H. Marshall, M. Fearnley, A. Holmes, and B. E. C. Nordin

The General Infirmary, Leeds, England

In a previous publication[1] we have confirmed the observation of Grodin *et al.*[2] that in a 3-day study about 3% of labelled androstenedione is converted to estrone in post-menopausal women, but we failed to show any significant correlation between conversion rate and age or body weight. Our data indicated that the major factor determining the post-menopausal plasma estrone concentration was the plasma concentration of androstenedione. We found that variations in conversion rates between individuals only exerted a small effect on the plasma estrone concentration. In the present study, we provide additional information about the relation between plasma androstenedione, plasma estrone and age in post-menopausal women.

Methods

Heparinized plasma samples were obtained in the fasting state from 15 peri-menopausal women, 50 women who had undergone a natural menopause, 20 oophorectomized women and 7 hysterectomized women attending our menopause clinic. The mean ages were 48, 58, 52 and 49 years respectively. Plasma estrone and androstenedione levels were measured by standard radioimmunoassay techniques using antisera obtained from Miles Laboratories Ltd and following their recommended procedure, with the important modification that only sodium dried ether was used for the extraction procedure. One ml of plasma was extracted into ether for the estrone assay and 0.5 ml for the androstenedione assay.

The plasma estrone levels in the 4 groups are shown in Figure 1.

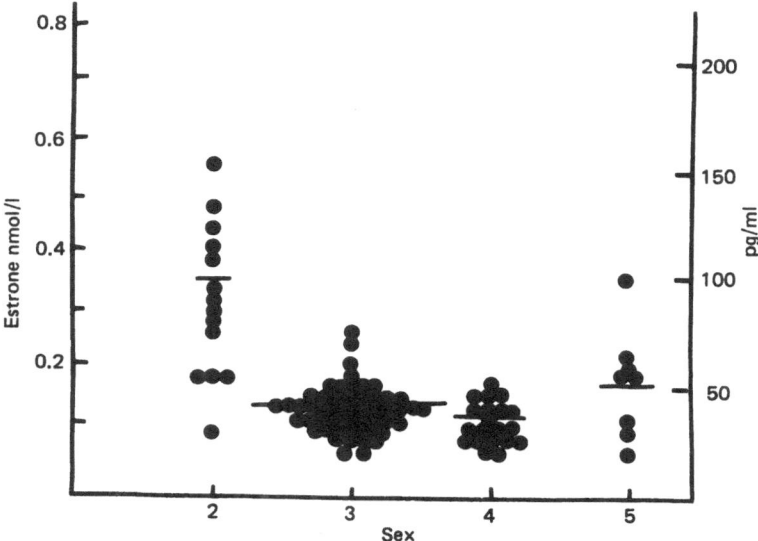

Figure 1   Plasma estrone levels in peri-menopausal women (sex 2), post-natural menopause (sex 3), post-oophorectomy (sex 4) and post-hysterectomy (sex 5)

The mean value is significantly higher in the peri-menopausal group (0.355 nmol/l) than in the other 3, which are not significantly different from each other. The corresponding androstenedione data are shown in Figure 2. The mean value is again significantly higher in the peri-menopausal group than in the 2 post-menopausal groups with the hysterectomized women falling in between, but there is a much greater overlap between pre- and post-menopausal women than in the estrone levels.

The relation between years since menopause and plasma estrone is shown in Figure 3. Apart from a few raised values within 2 years of the menopause in the natural menopause group, there is no obvious fall in plasma estrone with time elapsed since menopause in either group. However, statistical analysis shows that the mean plasma estrone in the post-natural group is significantly higher within 10 years of the menopause than it is later (Table 1). In the oophorectomized women this does not apply.

The corresponding androstenedione data are shown in Figure 4.

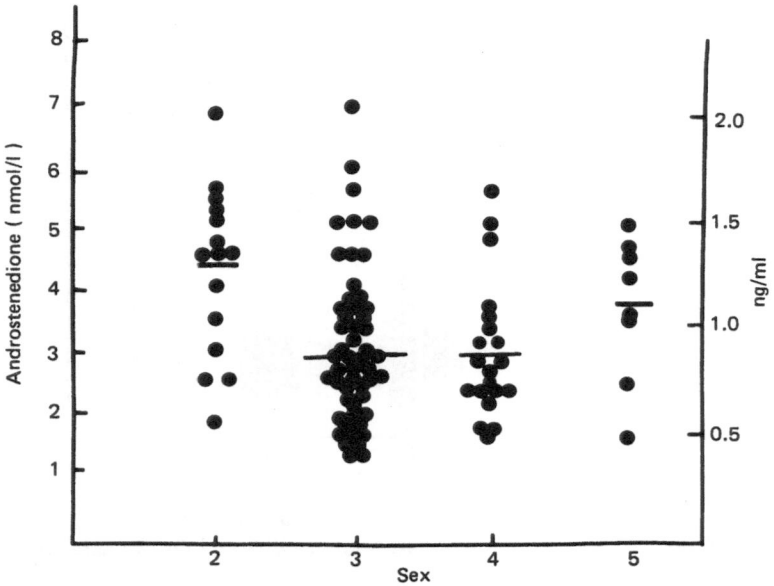

Figure 2   Plasma androstenedione levels in the same groups as Figure 1

It will be seen that there are some high values within 10 years of the menopause, mainly in the normal women, after which all the values are below 4 nmol/l. The mean value within 10 years of the menopause is 3.73 nmol/l in the post-natural group and 3.15 nmol/l in the oophorectomized group. Although this difference is not significant the oophorectomized mean is significantly lower than the peri-menopausal mean whereas the post-natural mean is not (Table 1). From 10 years on, the mean value is 2.42 nmol/l, and does not differ in the 2 groups.

Table 1   Estrone and androstenedione values (± 1 SE) with Student's t-test significances

Group	Number	Estrone (nmol/l)	Androstenedione (nmol/l)
Peri-menopausal	15	0.355 ± 0.045 $p < 0.001$	4.34 ± 0.36 NS
Natural menopause (YSM < 10)	25	0.138 ± 0.009 $p < 0.02$	3.73 ± 0.27 $p < 0.001$
Natural menopause (YSM ⩾ 10)	25	0.109 ± 0.006	2.34 ± 0.15
Oophorectomy (YSM < 10)	14	0.117 ± 0.008 NS	3.15 ± 0.32 NS
Oophorectomy (YSM ⩾ 10)	6	0.093 ± 0.013	2.77 ± 0.41

The correlation between the plasma androstenedione and estrone levels is shown in Figures 5, 6 and 7. Figure 5 shows that there is a very significant correlation between these variables in oophorectomized women, though the extrapolated regression line does not pass through the origin. Figure 6 shows a similar relationship in the post-natural menopause group but the estrone values tend to be above the mean regression line previously defined for the

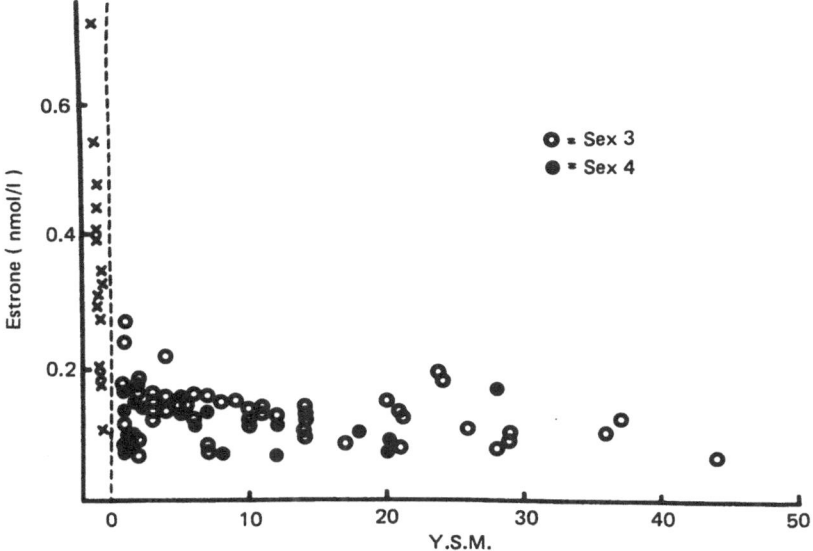

Figure 3   The relation between plasma estrone and years since menopause in the same groups as Figure 1. Hysterectomized women excluded

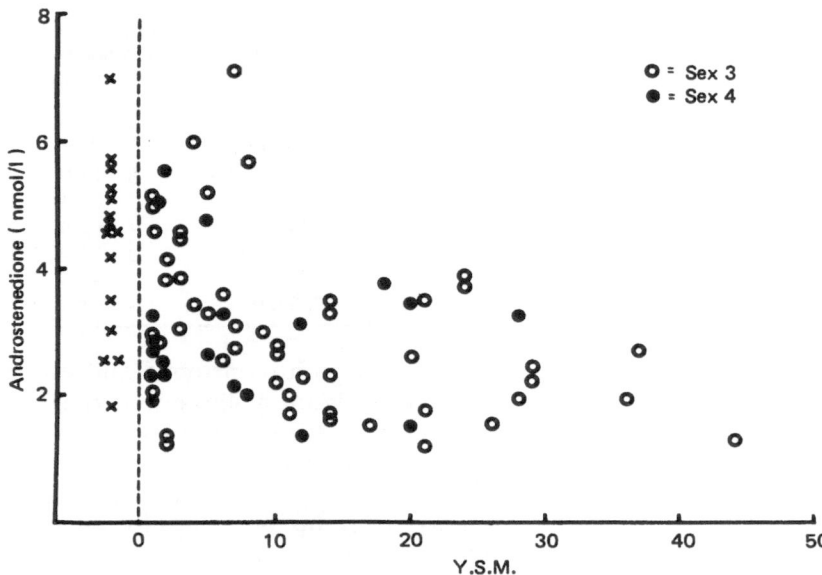

Figure 4 The relation between years since menopause and plasma androstenedione in the same cases as Figure 3

oophorectomized women. Figure 7 shows the corresponding relationship in the peri-menopausal and hysterectomized women. It is clear that in the former group the plasma estrone is much higher in absolute terms and relative to the plasma androstenedione than it is in the post-menopausal women. The data from the hysterectomized cases lie between the peri-menopausal and post-menopausal data.

Discussion

Our data confirm again the importance of androstenedione as the precursor of estrone in post-menopausal women and suggest again that the plasma androstenedione concentration, rather than the fractional rate of conversion to estrone, rises with age once the menopause has been passed. We suggest that the age effect reported by Grodin et al.[2] is simply due to the rise in conversion rate which seems to occur at the menopause. This rise may in fact be more apparent than real and simply follow from the fall in androstenedione level which occurs some years after the menopause (Figure 4). Since the extrapolated regression line of plasma estrone on androstenedione does not pass through the origin, but intersects the estrone axis at about 0.06 nmol/l, it follows that the estrone/androstenedione ratio (which presumably reflects the conversion rate) tends to be higher at lower values of androstenedione (Figures 5 and 6). At a plasma androstenedione of 7 nmol/l, the plasma estrone is 0.15 nmol/l or 2%; at an androstenedione level of 2 nmol/l the estrone is 0.9 nmol/l or 4.5%. Thus a fall in androstenedione level (as occurs some years after the menopause) is associated with an apparent rise in conversion rate which may simply reflect the kinetics of this enzyme-mediated reaction.

Our plasma estrone levels in pre- and post-menopausal women agree well with the results of other workers[3, 4] and their apparent constancy after the menopause is in accordance with the data of Longcope[3] who found no fall in plasma estrone with age in post-menopausal women. In fact, the prevailing estrone level in post-menopausal women is comparable to that in the follicular phase of pre-menopausal women. There is a tendency for the plasma estrone to be lower, in the first 10 post-menopausal years, in oophorectomized

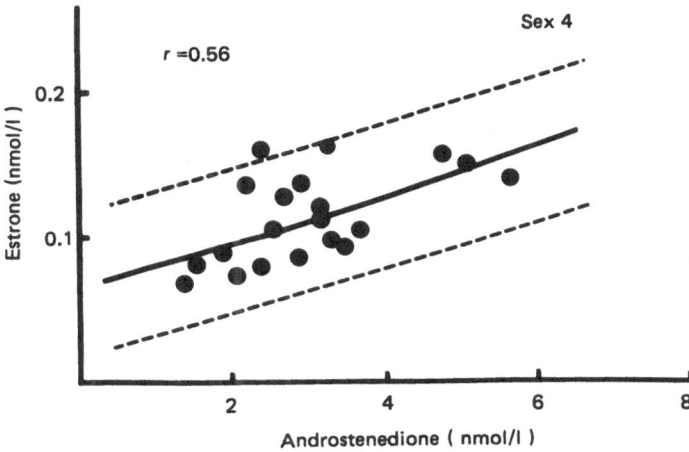

Figure 5 The relation between plasma androstenedione and plasma estrone in oophorectomized women

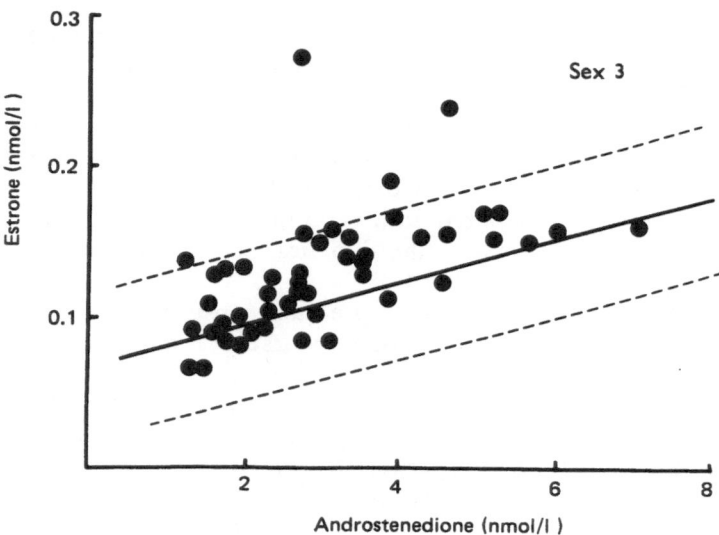

Figure 6 The relation between plasma androstenedione and plasma estrone in normal post-menopausal women, showing the regression line derived from Figure 5

women than in those who have gone through a natural menopause. This difference is significant and may indicate some residual estrone secretion by the post-menopausal ovaries, which continues for up to 10 years.

Our post-menopausal androstenedione levels also agree with those of other workers[5-7], but it is of interest to note that within 10 years of the menopause the mean value in the natural menopause group is higher than in the oophorectomized group (though not significantly) and significantly higher than it is later (Table 1). Moreover, the mean value of the natural menopause group within 10 years of the menopause is comparable with that of the peri-menopausal group, whereas the mean value in the oophorectomized cases is significantly lower than in the peri-menopausal ones. This confirms the idea that a substantial proportion (perhaps up to 50%) of the pre-menopausal plasma androstenedione derives from the ovaries[5], and that ovarian stromal secretion continues for up to 10 years after the cessation of

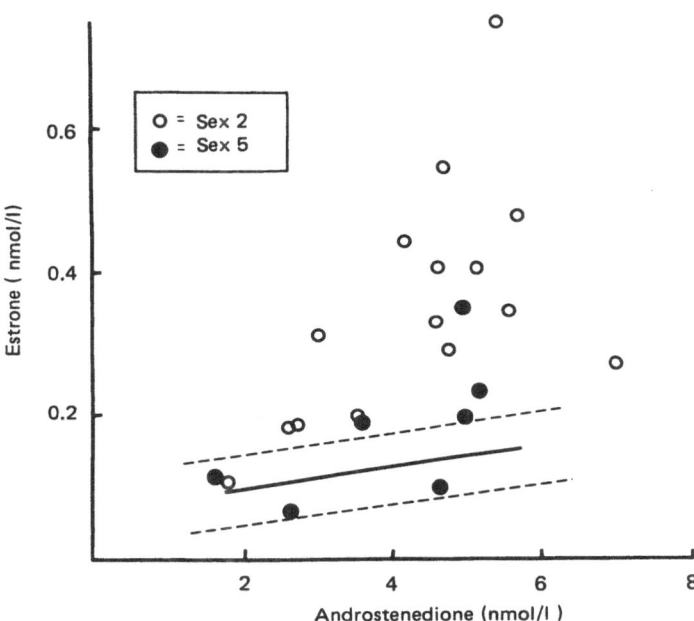

Figure 7 The relation between plasma androstenedione and plasma estrone in peri-menopausal and hysterectomized women. Regression lines as in Figures 5 and 6

menstruation in a proportion of normal women. This is also compatible with the data of Poortman *et al.*[6] which show the lowest androstenedione levels in the oldest post-menopausal women.

However, our peri-menopausal values tend to be lower than the values in young pre-menopausal women reported by other workers[4, 5, 8, 9]. Assuming that this is not due to technical differences, it seems that our peri-menopausal women with menopausal complaints and a mean age of 48 years have lower plasma androstenedione levels than normal, younger women, despite the fact that their estrone levels fall well within the young, pre-menopausal range. Does this mean that menopausal symptomatology is in part attributable to declining androstenedione production by the ovaries?

References

1. Pelc, B., Marshall, D. H., Nordin, B. E. C. and Khan, M. Y. (1976). Relation between plasma androstenedione, plasma oestrone and androstenedione to oestrone conversion rates in post-menopausal women. *Clin. Endocrinol.* (In press)

2. Grodin, J. M., Siiteri, P. K. and MacDonald, P. C. (1973). Source of oestrone production in post-menopausal women. *J. Clin. Endocrinol. Metab.*, **36**, 207

3. Longcope, C. (1974). Steroid production in pre- and post-menopausal women. *In: The Menopausal Syndrome.* (R. B. Greenblatt, V. B. Makesh and P. G. McDonough, editors) pp. 6–11. (New York, Medcom Press)

4. Makin, H. L. J. (1975). *Biochemistry of Steroid Hormones.* (Oxford, Blackwell Scientific Publications)

5. Abraham, G. E., Lobutsky, J. and Lloyd, C. W. (1969). Metabolism of testosterone and androstenedione in normal and ovariectomised women. *J. Clin. Invest.*, **48**, 696

6. Poortman, J., Thijssen, J. H. H. and Schwarz, F. (1973). Androgen production and conversion to estrogens in normal post-menopausal women and in selected breast cancer patients. *J. Clin. Endocrinol. Metab.*, **37**, 101

7. Judd, H. L., Judd, G. E., Lucas, W. E. and Yen, S. S. C. (1974). Endocrine function of the post-menopausal ovary: concentration of androgens and estrogens in ovarian and peripheral vein blood. *J. Clin. Endocrinol. Metab.*, **39**, 1020

8. Bardin, C. W. and Lipsett, M. B. (1967). Testosterone and androstenedione blood production rates in normal women and women with idiopathic hirsutism or polycystic ovaries. *J. Clin. Invest.*, **46**, 891

9. Baird, D. T., Burger, P. E., Heavon-Jones, G. D. and Scaramuzzi, Z. J. (1974). The site of secretion of androstenedione in non-pregnant women. *J. Endocrinol.*, **63**, 201

19

Influence of the Nutritional Status upon the Response of Menopausal Women to Estrogen Therapy

E. Vázquez, H. J. Casares* and J. A. Sereno†

Hospital Espanol, Mexico City, Mexico

Divergent results are sometimes encountered in patients similarly treated with estrogens to relieve menopausal symptoms and no evident explanation for them is usually mentioned, except for a vague reference to susceptibility, which amounts to not saying anything.

Our working hypothesis was that one possible reason for the apparently incoherent responses could be the nutritional status of the patients and/or their socioeconomic situation, which might influence the results—either through differences in receptors at the target organs, or through a different metabolism or turnover of the estrogen.

PATIENTS, MATERIALS AND METHODS

We selected three groups of post-menopausal patients in three separated geographical areas in Mexico, as follows:

Group I   : 34 patients of high income and good nutritional status, in Mexico City
Group II   : 30 patients of medium socioeconomic status, in Morelia
Group III: 20 patients of low income class, with deficient nutrition, in Mérida

In all three groups women were included who had severe menopausal symptoms which warranted hormonal therapy, who were at

*Hospital Regional de AMSS, Merida.   † Hospital Civil, Morelia.

least one year after the menopause and in whom pelvic and breast examination did not disclose any organic pathology. Papanicolaou smears were negative. Care was taken not to include women with a past history of liver disease or chronic alcoholism.

All patients were treated at the beginning with 2 mg of succinylestriol* *per os* daily. Each patient was seen at one month intervals to assess the development of symptoms and, if no improvement was obtained after 2 months, the dose was raised to 4 mg for 2 more months and then up to 6 mg daily if deemed necessary. The physical condition of the breasts and pelvic region, status of the skin, body weight and blood pressure were recorded at each visit.

A vaginal smear was taken in all patients at the end of 6 months. We also took endometrial biopsies at 6 months in selected patients on a randomized schedule, as follows: Group I: 19; Group II: 6; Group III: 15. To obtain a more accurate information on the estrogenic potency of succinylestriol throughout the treatment, we took an endometrial biopsy from ten patients of Group I at the end of the second month of treatment. Vaginal smears were simultaneously obtained.

The following liver function tests were performed on ten patients selected at random from each group: Direct and indirect bilirubin, alkaline phosphatase, pyruvic-oxaloacetic transaminase, bromsulphalein excretion, total plasma proteins and albumin/globulin ratio. They were repeated at the end of 6 months. As a second part of our study, 38 additional patients in the well-nourished group were treated with 2 mg of estradiol valerianate per day and studied in a similar way to those treated with succinylestriol.

RESULTS

The results obtained in the three groups of patients treated with succinylestriol differ from each other in several respects[1].

(a) *Vasomotor Symptoms*: Hot flushes and sweating were the most troublesome complaints, and their changes were taken as an index of efficacity of treatment. Their intensity was gauged and recorded from 0 (absent) to + + + (very severe). Table 1 shows that the low-income undernourished patients reported a more marked and earlier response to treatment, while those in the well-nourished group required more time and an increase in the dose of succinylestriol in most cases.

* This substance is also known as estriol succinate (Synapause)

Table 1   Results obtained in the treatment of vasomotor symptoms

	Group I	Group II	Group III
Improved, 1st cycle	6*	19*	17†
Improved, 2nd cycle	6*	10*	2†
Dose increased to 4 mg‡	9	—	—
Dose increased to 6 mg‡	7	—	—
Failures	6§	1	1§
TOTAL	34	30	20

* These patients received 2 mg daily
† These patients received 4 mg daily from the beginning
‡ These patients responded adequately to the increased dose
§ These are considered as failures because they did not respond even to the 6 mg
  dose

(b) *Metabolic Symptoms*: Backache, occipital headache which increases throughout the day and osteoarticular pains are the main
complaints of this type. Although they are sometimes difficult to
evaluate because they may be due to different causes, these symptoms
were relieved by the treatment in most patients. Since not all the
patients studied had symptoms of this kind, our results are expressed
as a common fraction in which the numerator represents the number
of patients who showed improvement and the denominator corres-
ponds to the total number of patients who complained of these
symptoms:

Group I   :   10/22
Group II :   16/22
Group III :   16/16

Among the patients in Group I and II who did not experience an
improvement in cephalalgia were some anxious and tense women,
whose headaches were most probably due to this reason rather than to
menopausal metabolic disturbances (osteoporosis).

Skin flaccidity and dryness were improved when these symptoms
were slight or moderate before starting the treatment, but no improvement was found when they were more marked. Expressed as a common fraction as above, the results were as follows:

Group I   :   7/14
Group II :   13/28
Group III :   4/8

There was no apparent effect on breast turgor, except for a doubtful improvement in one patient. Untoward effects such as engorgement, pain or tenderness were seldom noted. No masses or indurations were ever noticed at successive examinations.

(c) *Psychic Symptoms*: Anxiety, insomnia, irritability, depression and other symptoms of this kind were improved in a very irregular fashion. Insomnia was relieved when it was due mainly to hot flushes awakening the patient, but otherwise it needed somniferous drugs. Anxiety and depression went almost unchanged and required the help of a psychiatrist in a few cases.

(d) *Menstrual Disorders*: By definition all of our patients were between one and two years after the menopause, so there could be no changes in menstrual pattern. In no case were menses induced or restored; the few patients who had any bleeding during treatment are considered under the heading of undesirable effects.

(e) *Effects on the Vaginal Smear*: The effect of succinylestriol on the maturation of the vaginal wall as judged from smears was remarkable in the undernourished group, being most marked in those who had previously atrophic smears; this was apparent with the 2 mg-a-day dose. The least effect was obtained in the well-nourished group, in which the smear hardly showed any changes at the 2- and 4-mg levels, and it was only with the 6-mg dose that a maturation index of 40/30/30 was obtained.

(f) *Effect on the Endometrium*: Most endometria showed an atrophic pattern with the 2- and 4-mg doses after 6 months of therapy, but again there is a more marked effect in the undernourished patients than in the other groups, as shown in Table 2.

Table 2   Endometrial findings at the end of treatment

Type of endometrium	Group I	Group II	Group III
Early proliferative	6*	1	3
Late proliferative	3†	—	2
Hyperplastic	2	—	1
Atrophic	8	5	9

* Three of these patients were given 6 mg for the last two months
† These patients received 6 mg daily for the last two months

(g) *Effects on Liver Function Tests*: A remarkably uniform pattern was observed in this respect in all three groups of patients, for no significant change was demonstrated in any of the tests performed.

(h) *Undesirable Effects*: Under this heading we include those symptoms which were probably due to the steroid and were considered annoying or bothersome, Gastrointestinal complaints were completely absent and the drug was very well tolerated, Breast engorgement and slight soreness were mentioned by eight patients of the low-income group (at 2 mg a day) and by four patients in the well-nourished group (at the 6 mg a day). None of the patients in the intermediate group complained of breast discomfort at the 4 mg level.

Breakthrough bleeding was experienced by three patients in Group I, two in Group II and twelve in Group III. There was no dose–effect relationship but it is apparent that occurrence of this symptom was far more frequent in the poorly nourished women. No relationship was found between breakthrough bleeding and endometrial findings, nor was there any correlation between bleeding and the duration of therapy.

We obtained complete symptomatic relief in 30 out of the 38 patients treated with estradiol valerianate after 2 months of therapy and significant improvement was reported by four additional women. Our findings in endometrial biopsies and vaginal smears were basically similar to those found with 4–6 mg of succinylestriol and will be reported elsewhere.

DISCUSSION

The aim of any hormonal treatment is to cure and/or relieve symptoms of a particular condition, without disturbing other areas or causing undesirable effects ('secondary effects'), although they are strictly derived from the biological activity of the hormone. In the case of hormonal treatment of menopausal symptoms one aims at eliminating these without stimulating the endometrium or the breasts.

We can state from our results, that for all three groups of patients, succinylestriol is a compound capable of controlling in a satisfactory way the vasomotor symptoms of the climacteric in about 82% of women when given at a dose of 2–4 mg a day. This figure rises to 89% when the results of the 6 mg dose are included. However, we think that our data can be best interpreted if the results are analyzed for each group separately.

It was striking to see that if the low-income undernourished group plus the medium-income group are combined and separated from Group I, the proportion of improved cases with 2–4 mg of the steroid goes up to 96%, while the high-income patients show improvement in only 62% of the cases. Similar differences were found with the metabolic effects of the climacteric. One can speculate that the differences in response among the three groups of patients may well be due to changes either in the intermediate metabolism of the steroid which, according to van der Vies[2], is hydrolyzed by the liver upon gastrointestinal absorption, releasing free steroid into the blood stream. They may also be due to the number and effectiveness of specific receptors at the target organs.

As far as estrogenic potency is concerned, the endometrium and vaginal wall were more sensitive in the undernourished group and less sensitive in the high-income group. Our findings in this latter group show a negligible estrogenic stimulation, in agreement with previous reports[3]. The effect upon skin condition was very meager and only noted when dryness and atrophy were slight from the beginning; this agrees with previous reports with other steroids[4, 5]. Rauramo[6] has reported favourable structural changes in skin biopsies taken from castrated women treated with succinylestriol, and they were more intense after 6 than after 3 months. We found no demonstrable physical effect on the breasts at any dosage level.

Our results did not show any alteration in the liver function tests in any group, either at 2 or 6 months of treatment, in spite of the low protein ingestion in Group III. Cattoor et al.[3] reported a diminution in the bilirubin levels in plasma, for which no explanation could be found.

Undesirable effects were minimal and mostly negligible, the most common being slight breakthrough bleeding which amounted to spotting for 2 or 3 days and was more frequently found in the undernourished group. It did not require any treatment nor was it an indication for stopping the medication. No relationship was found between the endometrial biopsy and the presence of breakthrough bleeding, a fact that we find hard to explain at present.

Our findings on the additional group treated with estradiol valerianate show largely similar results, except that the 2-mg dose is more often effective than a similar dose of succinylestriol, a fact that was to be expected due to the difference in biological activity of the pure steroids from which the esters are derived. We do not think there is any relevant difference between the two compounds when each is given at an appropriate dose.

References

1. Vázquez, E. (1974). El climaterio. Concepto y manejo. *Rev. Fac. Med. (Méx.)*, **17**, 40
2. Van der Vies, J. (1968). Fate of oestriol-17-beta dihemisuccinate after oral administration to rats. *Acta Endocrinol. (Kbh)*, **48**, 630
3. Cattoor, J. P., Crabbé, G. and Engels, J. A. (1970). Utilisation du succinate d'oestriol dans la postmenopause. *Bruxelles-Med.*, **4**, 303
4. Davis, M. E. (1967). Estrogens and the retardation of ageing in post-menopausal women. In E. Gutiérrez Murillo and E.Vázquez (eds.) p. 307 (México). *Temas Selectos de Gineco-Obstetricia*
5. Greenblatt, R. B. (1955). Metabolic and psychosomatic disorders in menopausal women. *Geriatrics*, **10**, 165
6. Rauramo, L. (1969). Effets de la therapie oestrogenique par voie orale avec le succinate d'oestriol sur la peau des femmes castrées. *C.R. Soc. Fr. Gynecol.*, **39**, 327
7. Eisalo, A., Jarvinen, P. A. and Luukainen, T. (1965). Liver function tests during intake of contraceptive tablets in postmenopausal women. *Br. Med. J.*, **1**, 1416

20

Biochemical Parameters of Bone Metabolism in the Pre-, Peri-, and Post-menopausal State

H. C. van Paassen, S. A. Duursma,
J. M. M. Roelofs, J. v. d. Sluys Veer, R. Andriesse
and M. A. H. M. Wiegerinck

University Hospital, Utrecht, The Netherlands

INTRODUCTION

The suggestion of Albright *et al.*[1] in 1941 that osteoporosis is associated with the post-menopausal state has been sufficiently confirmed[2-5]. Kinetic studies, using [47]Ca and strontium, measuring the skeletal acretion rate of calcium, revealed normal values[6], whereas bone resorption was increased[7]. Significant differences in plasma calcium and phosphate between pre-menopausal women and women after natural or artificial menopause were published by Young *et al.*[8]. Gallagher *et al.*[9] showed a significant rise in the fasting plasma and urine calcium and phosphate levels after oophorectomy. The urinary hydroxyproline/creatinine ratio is higher in post-menopausal women than before menopause. Plasma alkaline phosphatase is known to be higher in women after the age of 50[11, 12].

Treatment with estrogens decreases plasma and urinary calcium and phosphate and a reduction in tubular reabsorption of phosphate is found[10]. Administration of estrogens causes a decrease in plasma alkaline phosphatase[13]. Bone resorption has been reduced by both androgens and estrogens, but after prolonged administration a decline in bone formation also occurs[7]. The aim of our investigation is to answer the following questions:

1. How is the sequence of the alterations in bone metabolism in the natural menopause?
2. Are the alterations in bone metabolism the result of a changed parathyroid function and/or of other influences.

The best method of investigation is a longitudinal study of the different parameters of bone metabolism. Before starting such a project a cross-sectional pilot study has been made. The results of this pilot study are presented in this paper.

MATERIAL AND METHODS OF INVESTIGATION

Ninety-one women, not receiving any hormonal agent (Group I), and 56 women, treated with different estrogen compounds (Group II) were investigated. The mean age of both groups was 51 years.

Subjects with oophorectomy or hysterectomy were excluded. All women were classified according to their menstrual age, by the method of Jaszmann[14]:

Group A: women menstruating regularly and women with a menstrual pattern similar to previous years.

Group B: women menstruating in the previous 12 months, but with a pattern different from the previous years.

Group C_1: women who had their last menstrual flow (L.M.) 1 to 2 years ago.

Group C_2: L.M. between 2 and 3 years ago.

Group C_3: L.M. between 3 and 4 years ago.

Group C_4: L.M. between 4 and 5 years ago.

Group C_5: L.M. between 5 and 10 years ago.

Group C_6: L.M. more than 10 years ago.

Plasma calcium, phosphate, alkaline phosphatase and parathyroid hormone concentration and the tubular reabsorption of phosphate as TmP/GFR[15] were determined in the fasting state. Calcium and phosphate excretion in urine were calculated as the mean of two values.

Calcium was determined by atomic absorption spectrophotometry; the inorganic phosphate was determined according to Fiske and Subarow; serum alkaline phosphatase was determined in accordance with Protocol 2409 of the Netherlands Institute for Standardization. Immunoreactive parathyroid hormone (iPTH) was determined by radio-immunoassay in the laboratory of Schopman and Hackeng in

Rotterdam. With this technique the whole hormone, the 1–34 fragment and a small number of other fragments are measured.

RESULTS

The mean values of the biochemical parameters for the different menstrual age groups are presented in Table 1. In the pre- and peri-

Table 1   Mean values ± SEM of bone parameters in menstrual age groups in women treated or untreated with estrogens

Menstrual age*		A	B	C_1	C_2+C_3	C_4+
	− estr.	28	13	6	9	35
	+ estr.	12	7	9	14	13
S. Ca	− estr.	2.52±0.02	2.53±0.04	2.56±0.02	2.58±0.02	2.57±0.02
(mmol/l)	+ estr.	2.52±0.03	2.52±0.04	2.54±0.04	2.60±0.04	2.52±0.03
	p	N.S.	N.S.	N.S.	N.S.	N.S.
S. P	− estr.	0.88±0.02	0.98±0.05	0.78±0.07	1.10±0.05	1.00±0.02
(mmol/l)	+ estr.	0.91±0.07	1.07±0.05	0.91±0.05	0.97±0.04	0.97±0.05
	p	N.S.	N.S.	< 0.05	< 0.025	N.S.
Ur. Ca	− estr.	4.4 ±0.5	5.0 ±0.5	4.3 ±0.7	6.8 ±1.2	4.3 ±0.3
(mmol/24 h)	+ estr.	4.5 ±0.8	4.6 ±0.5	4.3 ±0.4	4.5 ±0.5	4.1 ±0.8
	p	N.S.	N.S.	N.S.	< 0.05	N.S.
S. a. ph.	− estr.	55 ±3	54 ±5	67 ±7	81 ±5	72 ±3
(I.U./l)	+ estr.	52 ±4	64 +8	65 +6	67 ±5	70 ±4
	p	N.S.	N.S.	N.S.	< 0.05	N.S.
S. iPTH	− estr.	0.16±0.01	0.19±0.03	0.12±0.02	0.15±0.02	0.16±0.01
(ng/ml)	+ estr.	0.18±0.02	0.16±0.01	0.16±0.02	0.16±0.02	0.17±0.01
	p	N.S.	N.S.	N.S.	N.S.	N.S.
TmP/GFR	− estr.	0.92±0.04	1.02±0.07	0.68±0.07	1.18±0.09	0.97±0.04
(mmol/l)	+ estr.	0.93±0.11	1.05±0.07	0.95±0.08	1.01±0.04	0.91±0.05
	p	N.S.	N.S.	< 0.005	< 0.05	N.S.

* Menstrual age according to Jaszmann (1969)

menopausal women (Groups A and B) no difference exists between women with or without estrogen treatment. In Group C_1 the serum phosphate and TmP/GFR show a significant difference between treated and not-treated women. In $C_2 + C_3$ also calciuria and serum alkaline phosphatase are significantly higher in the untreated group. Untreated women more than 4 years post-menopausal, show a tendency to have higher values for serum calcium, phosphate and urinary calcium and TmP/GFR, than treated, but the differences are not significant.

Comparing the pre-(A) and post-menopausal (C_4+) groups (Table 2) no significant differences are observed for serum iPTH, urine calcium and TmP/GFR in both treated and untreated women. The women without therapy show a significantly higher serum calcium

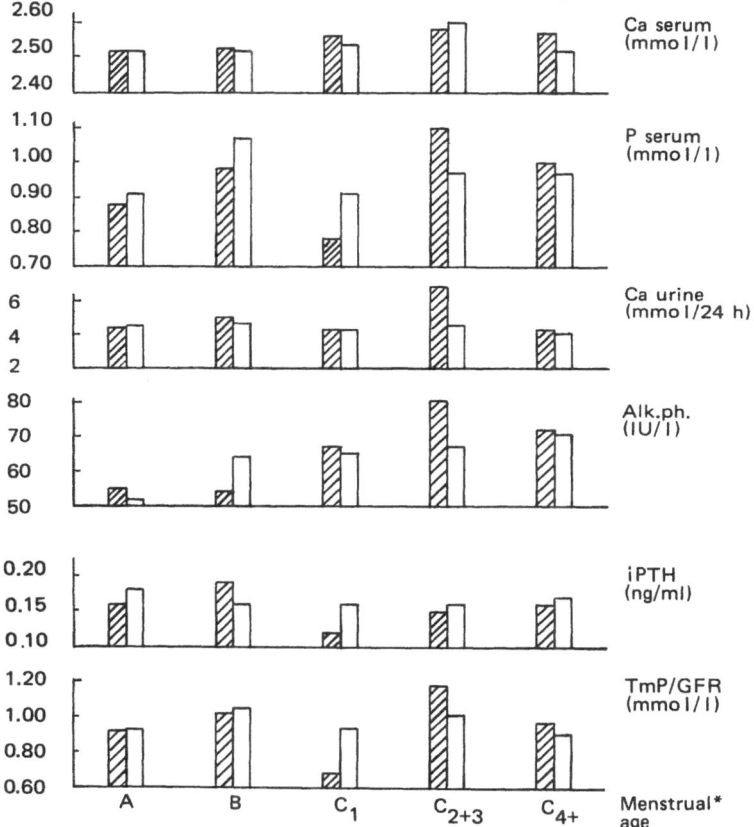

Figure 1 Data of bone metabolism in peri-menopausal women. Hatched columns: 91 women, no estrogen therapy; open columns: 56 women with estrogen therapy. (*Menstrual age according to Jaszmann[14])

and phosphate. Both treated and non-treated post-menopausal women show a significantly higher serum alkaline phosphatase than pre-menopausal women.

In Figure 1 the data are presented graphically.

Table 2 Mean values ± SEM of bone parameters in pre- and post-menopausal women treated or untreated with estrogens

Menstrual age*	Without estrogens			With estrogens		
	A $(n=28)$	C_4+ $(n=35)$	p value	A $(n=12)$	C_4+ $(n=13)$	p value
S. Ca (mmol/l)	2.52±0.02	2.57±0.02	<0.05	2.52±0.03	2.52±0.02	N.S.
S. P (mmol/l)	0.88±0.02	1.0 ±0.02	<0.001	0.91±0.07	0.97±0.05	N.S.
Ur. Ca (mmol/24 h)	4.4 ±0.5	4.3 ±0.3	N.S.	4.5 ±0.8	4.1 ±0.8	N.S.
S. a. ph (I.U./l)	55 ±3	72 ±3	<0.001	52 ±4	70 ±4	<0.005
S. iPTH (ng/ml)	0.16±0.01	0.16±0.01	N.S.	0.18±0.02	0.17±0.01	N.S.
TmP/GFR (mmol/l)	0.92±0.04	0.97±0.04	N.S.	0.93±0.11	0.91±0.05	N.S.

* Menstrual age according to Jaszmann (1969)

DISCUSSION

From cross-sectional investigation we get the impression that the first biochemical change is a rise in serum phosphate. In both treated and untreated women serum phosphate is higher in Group B than in Group A, significant at the 5% level. In the untreated women serum phosphate is lower in the following group (C_1), which is in accordance with the decrease of the TmP/GFR. In the next period $(C_2 + C_3)$ in treated and untreated persons nearly all parameters are higher than in the pre-menopause, the differences are more pronounced in the untreated persons. In this period the difference between the groups I and II (respectively without and with estrogen therapy) is significant for most of the parameters. Between the menstrual age groups with more than 4 years post-menopause $(C_4–C_6)$ we found no further differences.

Referring to our first question we have the impression from this cross-sectional study that the first change in bone metabolism is a rise in serum phosphate. Within a period of 3 years many secondary reactions take place and after 4 years apparently a new steady state has been reached. Although the women of Group II received estrogens the differences are not totally absent, but smaller than in non-treated women. For a correct view on the sequence of alterations a longitudinal study is necessary; the interval for examination of the women being no longer than half a year.

Some remarks about the mechanism can be made after comparing the data from period A and C_4+. The difference in serum alkaline phosphatase is highly significant in the untreated women. Alkaline phosphatase is an enzyme from liver and bone cells (osteoblasts) and in a small amount from the gut. The rise in serum alkaline phosphatase could be considered to be the result of an increase in bone turn-over. If this is a result of increased PTH-activity according to Heaney[1] and Nordin it should be combined with a lower TmP/GFR and serum phosphate. The results however point out that TmP/GFR and serum phosphate are higher, indicating a diminished PTH effect on the kidney.

Another possibility is that there is a dissociation of effects of PTH on bone and on kidney. This hypothesis can explain the tendency of serum phosphate, alkaline phosphatase and TmP/GFR to increase in combination with the unchanged level of iPTH. Possibly our radio-immunoassay for PTH is not sufficient to determine small differences or there may be a shift in the amounts of total hormone, 1–34 fragments and/or other fragments. A problem in this explanation may be why the raised serum calcium does not alter the PTH production. This problem may be explained by assuming that the higher level of serum calcium is for the larger part a dilutional effect[17].

Another way to explain the biochemical changes in the menopausal state can be considered, if one takes into account the interactions between estrogens and growth hormone. Growth hormone administration leads directly to a rise in TmP/GFR and serum phosphate[18]. By the way of growth hormone dependent serum sulphation factor it has also an action on bone[19]. Growth hormone and estrogens have an antagonistic effect on their target organs[20, 21]. A reduction of the estrogen level may result in an increased effect of growth hormone, which gives a rise in bone turn-over with release of calcium and phosphate from bone, and a rise in tubular reabsorption of phosphate in the kidney.

This mechanism can explain our data about serum calcium, phosphate, alkaline phosphatase and TmP/GFR. The results of this study suggest that the biochemical differences are more probably a result of a changed growth hormone effect than of a changed PTH effect.

References

1. Albright, F., Smith, P. H. and Richardson, A. M. (1941). Post-menopausal osteoporosis. Its clinical features. *J. Am. Med. Ass.*, **116**, 2465–2474

2. Meema, H. E. and Meema, S. (1968). Prevention of postmenopausal osteoporosis by hormone treatment of the menopause. *Can. Med. Ass. J.*, **99**, 248

3. Garn, S. M. (1970). The earlier gain and later loss of cortical bone. (Thomas, Illinois)

4. Davis, M. E., Lanzi, L. H. and Cox, A. B. (1970). Detection, prevention and retardation of postmenopausal osteoporosis. *Obstet. Gynaec. N.V.*, **36**, 187

5. Meunier, P., Coupron, P., Edourd, C., Bernard, J., Bringuier, J. and Vignon, E. (1973). Physiological senile involution and pathological rare fraction of bone. *Clin. Endocrinol. Metab.*, **2**, 239

6. Heaney, R. P. and Whedon, G. D. (1958). Radiocalcium studies of bone formation in human metabolic bone disease. *J. Clin. Endocrinol.*, **18**, 1246

7. Lafferty, F. W., Spencer, G. E. and Pearson, O. H. (1964). Effects of androgens, estrogens and high calcium intakes in bone formation and resorption in osteoporosis. *Am. J. Med.*, **36**, 514

8. Young, M. M., Nordin, B. E. C. (1967). Effects of natural and artificial menopause on plasma and urinary calcium and phosphorus. *Lancet*, **ii**, 118

9. Gallagher, J. C., Young, M. M. and Nordin, B. E. C. (1972). Effects of artificial menopause on plasma and urine, calcium and phosphate. *Clin. Endocrinol.*, **1**, 57

10. Gallagher, J. C. and Nordin, B. E. C. (1975). The effects of oestrogen and progestagen therapy on calcium metabolism in postmenopausal women. Oestrogens in the post menopause. *Front. Horm. Res.*, **3**, 157

11. Dequeker, J., Burssens, A., Creytens, G. and Bouillon, R. (1975). Ageing of bone in relation to osteoporosis and osteoarthrosis in postmenopausal women. In: van Keep en Lauritzen. Estrogens in the Post-Menopause. *Front. Horm. Res.*, **3**, 121

12. Klaassen, C. H. L. and Siertsma, L. H. (1964). De invloed van de leeftijd op de alkalische- fosfatase waarde n het serum. *Ned. Tijdschr. Geneeskd.*, **108**, 1433

13. Riggs, B. L., Jowsy, J., Kelly, P. J., Jones, J. D. and Maher, F. T. (1969). Effect of sex hormones on bone in primary osteoporosis. *J. Clin. Invest.*, **48**, 1065

14. Jaszmann, L., Lith, N. D. van, and Zaat, J. C. A. (1969). The perimenopausal symptoms. The statistical analysis of a survey. *Med. Gynaec. Social.*, **4**, 268

15. Bijvoet, I. L. M. and Sluys Veer, J. van der (1972). The assessment of phosphate reabsorption. *Clin. Endocrinol. Metab.*, **1:1**, 217

16. Heaney, R. P. (1965). A unified concept of osteoporosis. *Am. J. Med.*, **39**, 877

17. Aitken, J. M., Lindsay, R., Hart, D. M. (1974). The redistribution of body sodium in women on long term oestrogen therapy. *Clin. Sci. Mol. Med.*, **47**, 179

18. Corvilain, J. and Abramov, M. (1964). Effect of growth hormone on tubular transport of phosphate in normal and parathyroidectomized dogs. *J. Clin. Invest.*, **43**, 1608

19. Wiedemann, E. and Schwartz, F. (1972). Suppression of growth hormone dependent human serum sulfation factor by estrogen. *J. Clin. Endocrinol.*, **34**, 51

20. Schwartz, E., Wiedemann, E., Simon, S. and Schiffer, M. (1969a). Estrogenic antagonism of metabolic effects of administered growth hormone. *J. Clin. Endocrinol.*, **29**, 1176

21. Schwartz. E., Echemendia, E., Schiffer, M. and Panariello, V. (1969b). Mechanism of estrogenic action in acromegaly. *J. Clin. Invest.*, **48**, 260

22. Aitken, J. M., Gallagher, M. J. D., Hart, D. M., Newton, D. A. G. and Craig, A. (1973). Plasma growth hormone and serum phosphorus concentrations in relation to the menopause and to oestrogen therapy. *J. Endocrinol.*, **59**, 593

21

Effect of Long-Term Estrogen Therapy on Bone Remodelling in Women with a Natural Menopause: Cross-sectional and Longitudinal Study

J. Dequeker and J. Ferin

University of Louvain, Louvain, Belgium

INTRODUCTION

Bone metabolism data collected in a normal female population of all ages reveal remarkable differences between pre- and post-menopausal women[1]. Bone measurements indicate a loss of bone after the age of 50, due to increased bone resorption rather than to decreased bone formation[2]. Serum calcium and alkaline phosphatase activity rises after the menopause[2] as does the fasting urinary calcium: creatinine ratio[3].

The role of estrogens in these changes is not completely clear. In oophorectomized women a preventive effect of estrogen on bone loss has been shown in cross-sectional studies[4, 5] and has been confirmed in longitudinal studies[6, 7]. The extrapolation of the results in oophorectomized women to women with intact uteri is not justified.

The purpose of this study is to evaluate the effect of long-term estrogen treatment on bone mass and bone remodelling in women with a natural menopause.

METHODS

Cross-sectional Study

X-ray caliper measurements with a 0.1 mm readout of periosteal (D)

and endosteal (d) width of the right second metacarpal at midshaft were made on postero-anterior hand radiographs. The length of the second metacarpal was measured with millimeter rule. The cortical area values were calculated by subtracting the square of the endosteal diameter (d^2) from the square of the periosteal diameter (D^2). The values of periosteal and endosteal widths and cortical area were compared with sex specific norms as previously published[2, 8].

Longitudinal Study

For the longitudinal study a simplification of the method of Horsman and Simpson[9] was used in order to improve the reproducibility of the morphometric measurements. Pairs of hand films were measured blind by the same observer. For each pair of films, the averages over six metacarpals of periosteal width, endosteal width, cortical width and percentage cortical thickness were calculated. The reproducibility of the method has been evaluated using the measurements of six post-menopausal women, who had three pairs of hand radiographs taken the same day. The coefficients of variation obtained by using the mean values of six metacarpals are considerably better than those obtained by measuring one metacarpal (Table 1). For longitudinal studies the evaluation of the mean of six metacarpals is to be preferred.

Table 1   Comparison of coefficients of variation between measurements obtained at one metacarpal (second) and obtained in six metacarpals

	Second metacarpal		Six metacarpals	
Periosteal diameter (D)	1.68	±0.60	0.82	±0.37
Endosteal diameter (d)	3.77	±2.16	2.23	±1.27
Cortical thickness $(D-d)$	3.09	±1.65	1.29	±0.40
% cortical thickness $(D-d/D)$	2.23	±1.03	0.91	±0.14

SUBJECTS

Cross-sectional Study

Eighty-five women with a natural menopause, age range 47–72 years, received long-term estrogen replacement therapy with either conjugated equine estrogen 1.25 mg or ethinyl estradiol 0.025 mg daily, with at intervals of 4–6 weeks a short course of progestogen.

Treatment was started in all patients within 1 year after cessation of menstruation. Only those who had replacement for more than 2 years were included. All subjects were more than 45 years old at the time when the hand X-ray was taken. Duration of treatment was in 35 subjects 2–4.9 years, in 31 subjects 5–9.9 years and in 19 more than 10 years.

Twenty-nine women with a natural menopause of the same practice, age range 46–69 years, who received no replacement therapy served as controls.

Longitudinal Study

A total of 29 women, who had a natural menopause, age range 42–61 years, were evaluated. All subjects received during the follow-up continuously conjugated equine estrogen 1.25 mg daily. The follow-up period varied from 12 months up to 38 months, mean 21.5 months. Twenty-five of them were already on estrogen replacement therapy, mean 4.5 years ± 4.4, which was started within one year after cessation of the menstruation. Four subjects, who had their menopause within the last 2 years, started their replacement therapy at the start of the study.

RESULTS

Cross-sectional Study

The values of periosteal diameter, endosteal diameter and cortical area of the second metacarpal at midshaft obtained in 85 estrogen treated post-menopausal women and in 29 untreated post-menopausal women are shown in Figure 1. The mean values of the sex-specific control group are represented by the broken lines. The periosteal-, endosteal-diameter and bone mass of the untreated group are evenly distributed on both sides of the normative trend line, as are the values of the periosteal diameter of the estrogen treated group. The distribution of the endosteal diameter values in the estrogen treated group differs significantly from the control group. Treated women had a below average endosteal diameter, indicating reduced resorption.

The distribution of cortical area values in treated post-menopausal women differs significantly from the control group. Treated women

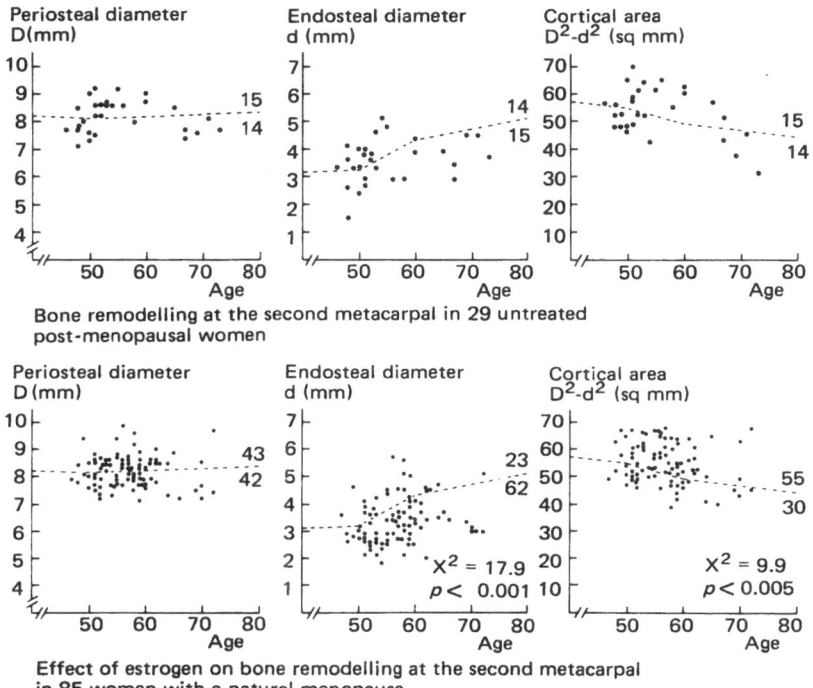

Figure 1 Bone remodelling at the second metacarpal in 29 untreated and 85 estrogen treated women with a natural menopause

had a larger bone mass than expected and this remained statistically significant even after more than 10 years treatment.

Longitudinal study

In Figure 2 are plotted the values of percent difference before and after therapy in periosteal diameter, endosteal diameter, cortical thickness and percent cortical thickness in 29 post-menopausal women on conjugated equine estrogen. The dashed lines indicate the error range and the full line the mean change and SD over a period of 24 months for 20 untreated post-menopausal women.

No significant changes in periosteal-, endosteal-diameter and cortical thickness occurred during the follow-up period in the estrogen treated women and in periosteal diameter in the untreated women.

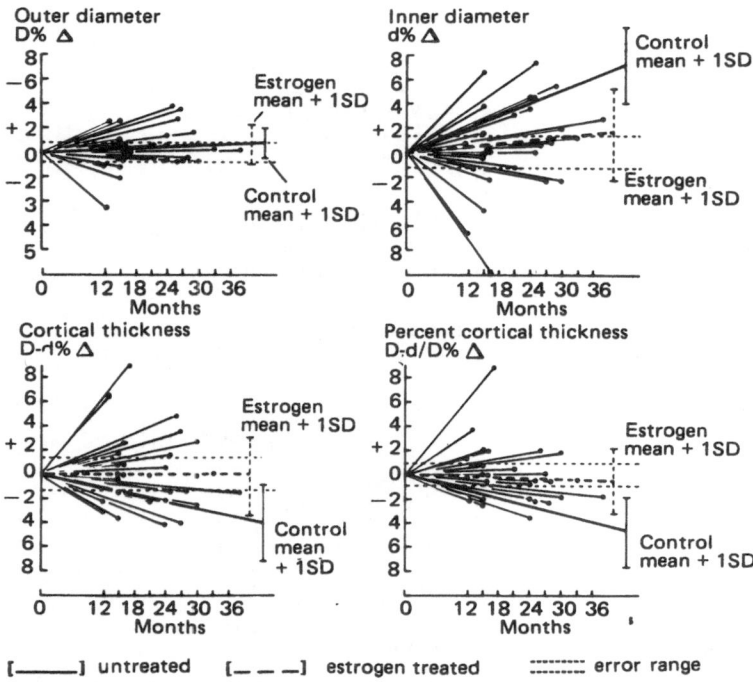

Figure 2 Sequential changes in cortical bone of estrogen treated post-menopausal women compared to mean values of cortical bone remodelling of untreated post-menopausal women

Table 2   Mean age and mean percent change and SD in metacarpal bone during follow-up period in 20 untreated menopausal women compared to 29 estrogen treated post-menopausal women

	No treatment		*Estrogen treatment*			
	mean	SD	mean	SD	*t*	*P*
Number	20		29			
Age	55.3	±4.7	53.3	±5.0	+1.397	n.s.
Outer diameter % difference	100.4	±1.2	100.4	±1.6	+0.025	n.s.
Inner diameter % difference	104.4	±3.7	100.6	±3.8	+3.646	*p* < 0.001
Cortical thickness % difference	97.5	±3.3	100.1	±3.1	−2.697	*p* < 0.02
% Cortical thickness % difference	97.2	±2.9	99.8	±2.5	−3.420	*p* < 0.005

In the untreated group the endosteal diameter increased, while the cortical thickness decreased during the follow-up period. In the estrogen treated group there was no increase in endosteal diameter, with as a result no change in cortical thickness or percent cortical thickness. The difference in mean changes in endosteal diameter, cortical thickness and percent cortical thickness between the untreated and treated group is statistically significant (Table 2).

DISCUSSION

Bone remodelling in estrogen-treated menopausal women differs from normal controls matched for age and sex by a lower endosteal bone resorption rate with, as a result, a significantly larger bone mass than untreated control subjects. The results of the study are in good agreement with the reports on estrogen treatment in oophorectomized women of Davis et al.[4], who used a finger-bone mineral densitometry method and of Meema and Meema[5], who used the simple cortical thickness measurement of the radius. Aitken et al.[6] in a double blind controlled mestranol trial found with a photon absorption technique a prevention of bone loss at the second metacarpal bone in oophorectomized women.

The subjects of this study differ from those of other reports by the fact that all subjects had a natural menopause, and thus a less precise menopausal period and an intact uterus, which may be a reason for intermittent therapy, in order to ensure regular shedding of the endometrium. In spite of this handicap estrogen therapy started within 1 year after cessation of menstruation in women with a natural menopause is effective as shown in this cross-sectional and longitudinal study.

The radiogrammetry method of measuring bone mass derived from metacarpal periosteal and endosteal diameter at midshaft has the advantage of giving information on bone remodelling processes and thus on the mechanism by which the estrogen therapy influence bone mass. Estrogen prevents bone loss by reducing endosteal bone loss and not by increasing bone apposition at the periosteal surface. The longitudinal data showed that the untreated group lost bone at a rate of 1.15% per year and that conjugated equine estrogen treatment prevented this bone loss by inhibiting endosteal bone resorption.

The preventive effect of estrogen is not of short duration since this effect could be demonstrated in patients who were already on long-term estrogen therapy before the first evaluation. This finding is at variance with that of Riggs *et al.*[10, 11], who found a temporary effect in women with compressed vertebrae on long-term equine conjugated estrogen of 42 months.

The present results obtained in a homogenous cross-sectional and longitudinal study give support to the prophylactic treatment of osteoporosis by estrogen in post-menopausal women with intact uteri. The prolonged administration of estrogen, conjugated equine estrogen or ethinyl estradiol appeared to be reasonably safe since no serious deleterious effects have been observed in this group (Ferin and Thomas 1973)[12].

SUMMARY

The effect of long-term estrogen treatment on bone remodelling and bone mass at the metacarpal bone was studied in 114 women with a natural menopause.

Cross-sectional data were collected in 85 and longitudinal data in 29 post-menopausal women. The data were compared with values obtained in untreated post-menopausal women.

Bone mass decreased and endosteal resorption increased significantly in the untreated women. The untreated group lost bone at a rate of 1.15% per year. Bone remodelling in estrogen treated women with a natural menopause differs from normal controls matched for age by a lower endosteal bone resorption rate with as a result a significant larger bone mass than untreated control subjects. The effect of estrogen was not temporary since the beneficial effect could be demonstrated in women who had a replacement therapy for more than 10 years.

The present results obtained in a homogenous group of women with a natural menopause support the prophylactic treatment of osteoporosis by estrogen in post-menopausal women with intact uteri.

References

1. Dequeker, J., Burssens, A., Creytens, G. and Bouillon, R. (1975). Ageing of bone: its relation to osteoporosis and osteoarthrosis in post-menopausal women. *Front. Horm. Res.*, **3**, 116
2. Dequeker, J. (1972). *Bone Loss in Normal and Pathological Conditions*. p. 214 Leuven University Press,

3. Nordin, B. E. C., Gallagher, J. C., Aaron, J. E. and Horsman, A. (1975). Postmenopausal osteopenia and osteoporosis. *Front. Horm. Res.*, **3**, 131
4. Davis, M. E., Strandjord, N. M. and Lanzl, L. H. (1966). Estrogens and the aging process. *J. Am. Med. Ass.*, **196**, 219
5. Meema, H. E. and Meema, S. (1968). Prevention of postmenopausal osteoporosis by hormone treatment of the menopause. *Can. Med. Ass. J.*, **99**, 248
6. Aitken, J. M., Hart, D. M. and Lindsay, R. (1973). Oestrogen replacement therapy for prevention of osteoporosis after oophorectomy. *Br. Med. J.*, **2**, 515
7. Meema, S., Bunker, M. L. and Meema, H. E. (1975). Preventive effect of estrogen on postmenopausal bone loss: A follow-up study. *Arch. Intern. Med.*, **135**, 1436
8. Dequeker, J. (1971). Periosteal and endosteal surface remodelling in pathological conditions. *Invest. Radiol.*, **6**, 260
9. Horsman, A., Simpson, M. (1975). The measurement of sequential changes in cortical geometry. *Br. J. Radiol.*, **48**, 471
10. Riggs, B. L., Jowsey, J., Kelly, P. J., Jones, J. D. and Maher, F. T. (1969). Effect of sex hormones on bone in primary osteoporosis. *J. Clin. Invest.*, **48**, 1065
11. Riggs, B. L., Jowsey, J., Goldsmith, R. S., Kelly, P. J., Hoffman, D. L. and Arnaud, C. D. (1972). Short- and long-term effects of estrogen and synthetic anabolic hormone in postmenopausal osteoporosis. *J. Clin. Invest.*, **51**, 1659
12. Ferin, J. and Thomas, K. (1973). Long-term replacement therapy in postmenopausal women. *Front. Horm. Res.*, **2**, 134

22

The Effect of Castration and Oral Estrogen Therapy on Serum Lipids

R. Punnonen and L. Rauramo

University of Turku, Turku, Finland

The serum cholesterol level in pre-menopausal women is lower than in men of the same age. A correlation between the serum cholesterol level and coronary disease has been demonstrated, and before the age of 40 years coronary disease is also distinctly less common in women than in men. After the menopause these differences between the sexes soon become less pronounced and disappear. It was hoped that estrogen therapy would prevent the increase of serum lipids and possibly prevent and slow down the development of coronary disease. The effects of long term estrogen therapy are therefore of particular interest. The purpose of the present study was to clarify the effects of castration and oral estriol succinate and estradiol valerate therapy on serum cholesterol, triglyceride and phospholipid levels.

SUBJECTS AND METHODS

Bilateral oophorectomy was usually performed in association with hysterectomy for uterine myomas. The effect of castration on serum cholesterol, triglycerides and phospholipids was investigated in 100 women with a mean age of 48 years. All patients had menstruated up to the time of operation. The lipid levels were investigated pre-operatively and one month after castration.

The estrogen therapy employed was estriol succinate at a dose of 2 mg/day. The 50 women (mean age 48 years) received this therapy uninterruptedly over a period of 3 years. The therapy was started 1 month after castration. Serum lipids were investigated in these patients after 3 months and thereafter every 6 months. In addition serum lipids were checked in 10 patients (mean age 48 years) preoperatively and 3 years postoperatively.

One month after operation oral estradiol valerate treatment at a dose of 2 mg/day was started in 25 patients (mean age 48 years). This treatment was continued for a period of 6 months. Serum lipids were investigated after 6 month's estrogen therapy. The control group comprised 25 patients (mean age 49 years), who did not receive estrogen therapy after castration.

Blood samples for the lipid determinations were taken after overnight fasting. The serum cholesterol levels were determined according to Pearsson et al.[1] (normal values 4.1–7.7 mmol/l), triglycerides by the Royer and Ko method[2] (normal values 0.4–1.7 mmol/l) and phospholipids according to Bartlett[3] (normal values 2.6–4.1 mmol/l).

RESULTS

Castration. The preoperative serum cholesterol level was 6.8 ± 0.1 mmol/l and a month after castration 7.3 ± 0.2 mmol/l. The corresponding triglyceride values were 1.2 ± 0.1 mmol/l and 1.4 ± 0.1 mmol/l respectively and phospholipids 3.4 ± 0.1 and 3.7 ± 0.1 mmol/l (100 patients). All these differences are statistically significant ($p < 0.05$).

Estriol Succinate Therapy. Figure 1 shows the cholesterol level of patients treated with estriol succinate over a period of 3 years (Figure 1). Shortly after the start of the therapy the cholesterol level showed no further increase. After about $1\frac{1}{2}$ years of estriol succinate therapy the cholesterol level showed a tendency to decrease. The changes in serum triglyceride level were minimal during estriol succinate therapy. At the beginning of the therapy the triglyceride level was 1.4 ± 0.1 mmol/l, and 1.3 ± 0.1 mmol/l after the 3 years therapy (Figure 2). The phospholipid levels also failed to show significant changes (Figure 3). In the control group (10 patients) the serum cholesterol tended to rise during the 3 years. The changes in the triglycerides and phospholipids were minimal (Figure 4).

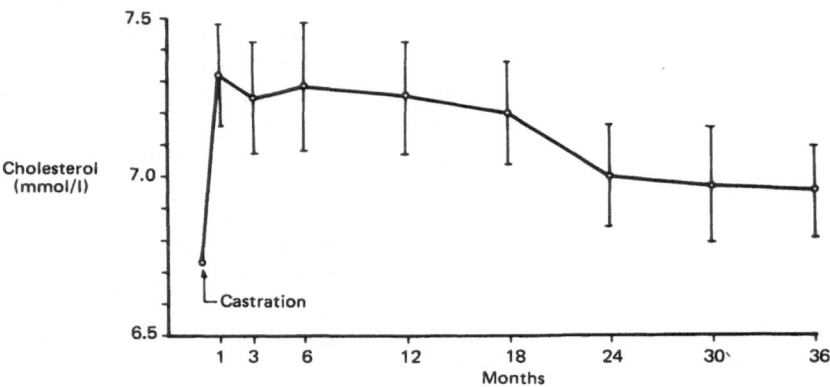

Figure 1   Effect of oral estriol succinate therapy on serum cholesterol

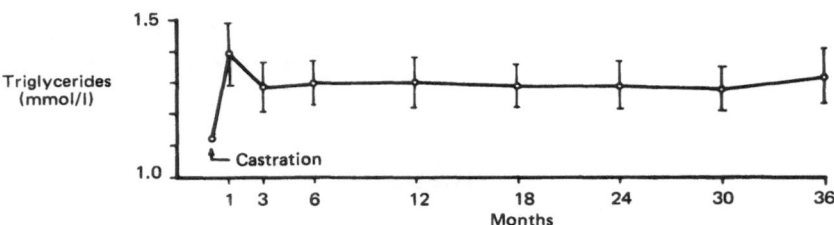

Figure 2   Effect of oral estriol succinate therapy on serum triglycerides

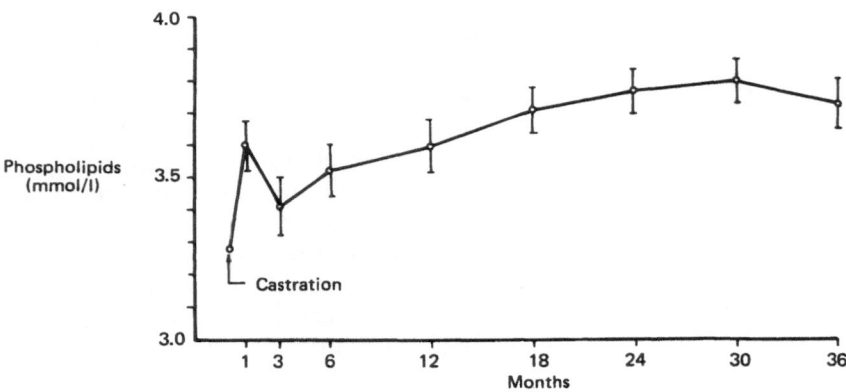

Figure 3   Effect of oral estriol succinate therapy on serum phospholipids

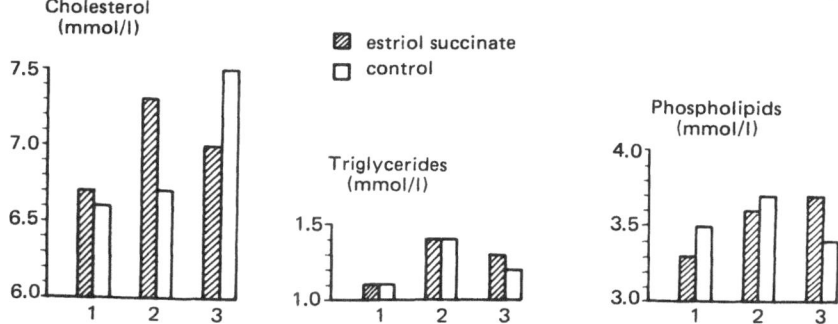

Figure 4 Effect of estriol succinate therapy and bilateral oophorectomy (control) on serum cholesterol, triglycerides and phospholipids. 1. Before operation, 2. 1 month after operation, 3. 3 years after operation

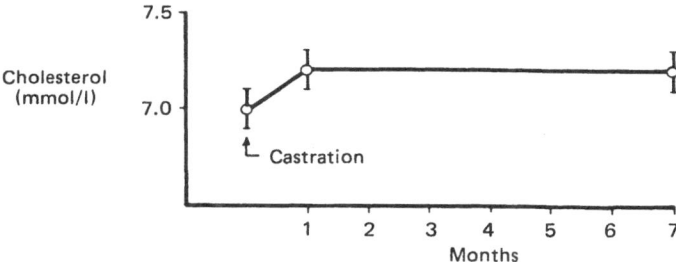

Figure 5 Effect of oral estradiol valerate therapy on serum cholesterol

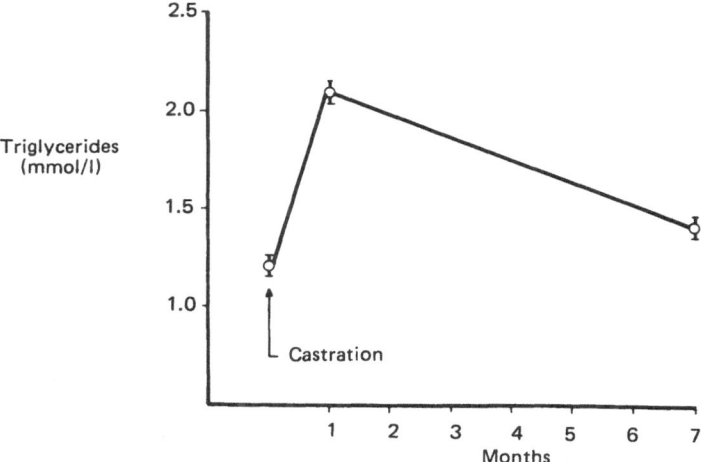

Figure 6 Effect of oral estradiol valerate therapy on serum triglycerides

Estradiol valerate therapy. The cholesterol level remained almost unchanged during the 6 months treatment (Figure 5). In the control
group (without hormone therapy) the cholesterol showed a slight
tendency to rise. The triglyceride level showed a tendency to decrease
during estradiol valerate therapy. At the start of the therapy the triglyceride level was 2.1 ± 0.1 mmol/l and 1.4 ± 0.1 mmol/l after the 6
months treatment (Figure 6). These values did not differ significantly
from the control group. The phospholipid level increased from $3.7 \pm$
0.1 to 4.0 ± 0.4 mmol/l ($p < 0.05$) (Figure 7). There were no significant
changes in the control group.

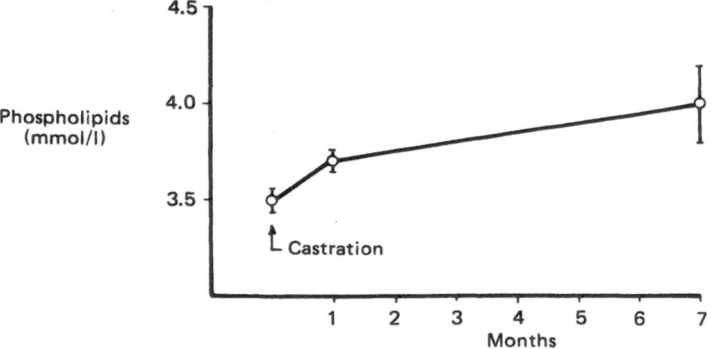

Figure 7   Effect of oral estradiol valerate therapy on serum phospholipids

DISCUSSION

After a natural menopause the ovaries may still secrete estrogens. All
the patients studied had been castrated and errors caused by endogenous estrogen excretion were therefore minimal. The mean age of
the groups treated with estrogens and that of the control group is
similar. The time interval between castration and the start of the
estrogen therapy was the same for all patients (1 month).

In the present study the serum cholesterol, triglyceride and phospholipid levels showed a significant rise 1 month after castration. In
many studies estrogens have been shown to increase serum triglycerides. In theory, the effect of castration should be to cause a decrease
rather than an increase of the triglyceride level. That this is not the
case is apparently due to the cyclic estrogen–progesteron excretion in
menstrual women. The cyclic increase of progesterone levels nor-

malizes the elevation of the triglycerides that occurs during the estrogen dominance.

Julesz and co-workers[4] showed that small doses of estriol affect lipid metabolism. The effect of long term estriol therapy on the serum lipids has not previously been investigated. In the present study the serum cholesterol showed no further increase after the start of the estriol succinate therapy, and after $1\frac{1}{2}$ years it showed a tendency to decrease. In the control group the cholesterol level tended to rise during the 3 years after operation. Numerous trials[5, 6] have shown that estrogens increase the serum triglyceride level. In the present study the level remained almost unchanged during estriol succinate therapy lasting 3 years. Besides cholesterol, a correlation has also been found between the serum triglyceride level and coronary disease. The changes in serum phospholipid level were minimal.

Many investigations have demonstrated that estrogens increase the serum phospholipid level. It has been suggested that the serum phospholipids may act as cholesterol stabilizers and the relative deficiency of phospholipids may contribute to the accumulation of cholesterol in the tissues.

During the 6 months estradiol valerate therapy the cholesterol level remained virtually unchanged. There were no significant differences between the patients treated with estradiol valerate and the control group. It must be taken into consideration however, that the serum cholesterol levels were in the normal range at the start of both estriol succinate and estradiol valerate therapy and any possible cholesterol lowering effect would be poorly demonstrated.

SUMMARY

The effect of castration on serum lipids was studied in 100 women (mean age 48 years). Serum cholesterol, triglyceride and phospholipid levels showed a significant ($p < 0.05$) increase one month after castration. The estrogen therapy employed in the 50 women (mean age 48 years) was estriol succinate at a dose of 2 mg/day and the treatment was started 1 month after castration and continued for 3 years. At the end of the treatment the cholesterol level showed a tendency to decrease and in the control group a corresponding tendency to rise. The changes in serum triglyceride and phospholipid levels during estriol succinate therapy of 3 years duration were minimal. The estrogen therapy employed in 25 women (mean age 48 years) was estradiol valerate 2 mg/day over a period of 6 months. At the end of this therapy the phospholipid level had increased significantly ($p < 0.05$). Also during the estradiol valerate therapy the changes in cholesterol and triglyceride levels were minimal.

References

1. Pearson, S., Stern, S. and McGavack, T. (1953). A rapid accurate method for the determination of total cholesterol in serum. *Anal. Chem.*, **25**, 813
2. Royer, M. E. and Ko, H. (1969). A simplified semiautomated assay for plasma triglycerides. *Anal. Biochem.*, **29**, 405
3. Bartlett, G. R. (1959). Phosphorus assay in column chromatography. *J. Biol. Chem.*, **234**, 466
4. Julesz, M., Fröhlich, M. B., László, I. K., Tóth, I., Szepessy, G. and Dávid, M. A. (1963). Uber die Wirkung des Oestriols auf den Lipoidstoffwechsel. *Acta Med. Acad. Sci. Hung.*, **29**, 161
5. Punnonen, R. and Rauramo, L. (1976). Effect of bilateral oophorectomy and peroral estradiol valerate therapy on serum lipids. *Int. J. Gynaecol. Obstet.*, **14**, 13
6. Punnonen, R. and Rauramo, L. (1976). Effect of castration and long-term oral estrogen therapy with estriol succinate on serum lipids. *Ann. Chir. Gynaecol. Fenn.*, **65**, 216

23

Experience with Endometrial Irrigations in Menopausal Women

M. J. Casey and T. J. Madden

University of Connecticut School of Medicine,
Connecticut, USA

INTRODUCTION

The use of estrogens for contraception, treatment of peri-menopausal symptoms and induction of end-organ effects has proliferated within the past 20 years, and the benefits derived from the use of these drugs have been outstanding. Whether or not estrogenic drugs, increasing longevity with decreasing mortality from other diseases or other environmental factors are responsible for the apparent increased incidence of endometrial carcinoma which has been seen in Connecticut, the burden of responsibility for diagnosis of this disease in its earliest, most curable stages, is upon the practising physician and public health officials.

Since 1972, we have been evaluating the negative pressure endometrial irrigator for its feasibility as a screening technique in asymptomatic women. The experience we have gained with this method is the subject of our report.

METHODS AND MATERIALS

The device and technique for negative pressure jet-irrigation of the endometrial cavity have been described[1]. We have experience with over 300 endometrial irrigations. More than 250 of these have been done using aseptic technique on unanaesthetized patients between 32 and 80 years of age. Following preparation and sounding of the uterine cervix the irrigator tip was introduced and lavage was carried out with 30–40 ml of sterile normal saline solution. The irrigant was fixed by adding equal amounts of 70% ethanol. Gross tissue fragments were removed and submitted for histological study. The fluid was then divided into two parts. The first aliquot was centifuged and the sediment prepared for cytological study by the Papanicolaou technique prior to paraffin imbedding for routine histological sections. The second aliquot was passed through a 5 micron Millipore filter and then stained by the Papanicolaou technique for cytological study. Cytological examination was supported by direct cervico-vaginal smear, smear of the centifuged sediment and the filter preparation; whereas the histological study was carried out on the gross tissue fragments and cell block preparation of the centifuged sediment.

Prior to surgical dilation of the cervix and curettage of patients undergoing general anaesthesia for clinical indications, endometrial irrigations were carried out and the tissues obtained were compared with the endometrial curettings. Over 225 successful irrigations have been carried out on asymptomatic women without anaesthesia. Two-hundred and one successive attempted endometrial irrigations on asymptomatic women over 40 years of age were the subject of a special study of patient and physician acceptance of these techniques and adequacy for cytohistological diagnosis[2].

Material obtained by negative pressure curettage of the endometrial cavity using the Vabra aspirator on anaesthetized and unanaesthetized patients has been examined using routine histological processing.

Twenty-five gynaecologists associated with the University of Connecticut have taken part in this study.

RESULTS

Cytohistology

The endometrial irrigation technique has been highly successful in obtaining material adequate for cytological and histological evaluation. Figure 1 is a microphotograph of normal tall columnar endocervical cells on a filter preparation from a post-menopausal

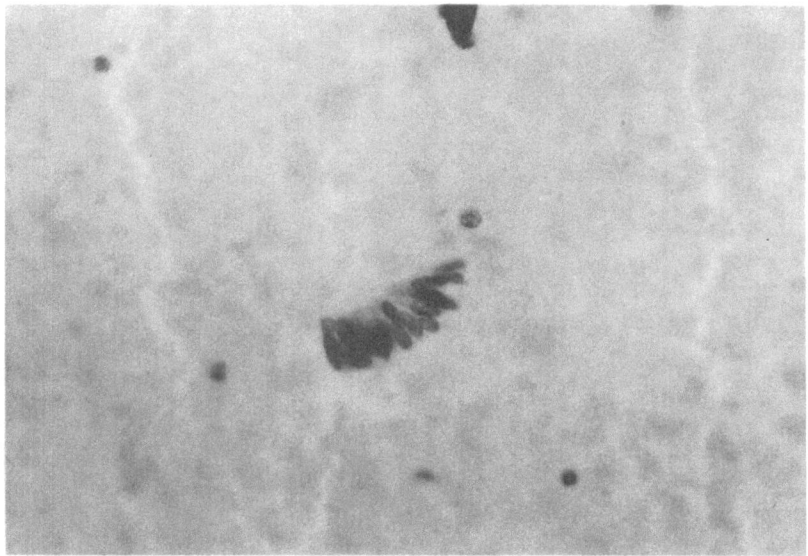

Figure 1   Tall columnar endocervical cells. High power. Filter preparation

woman. Figure 2 illustrates normal endometrial glandular cells from a post-menopausal female. These cells are uniform in size and have finely granular nuclei with pale scanty cytoplasm. Benign endometrial glandular cells frequently occur in clusters, but increasingly severe endometrial pathology is associated with increasing numbers of endometrial cells and cell clumps. Cells on a filter preparation from endometrial irrigation of a post-menopausal woman with well differentiated adenocarcinoma of the endometrium are shown in Figure 3. Note the irregularity in cell size and nuclear-cytoplasmic ratio; coarse chromatin and prominent multiple nucleoli may be present. Figure 4 is an example of the histology of well differentiated endometrial adenocarcinoma seen in a cell block preparation of a uterine irrigation.

Cytohistological interpretation of the specimens prepared from endometrial lavages was highly accurate in the diagnosis of adenocarcinoma of the endometrium. In a study of 40 mildly symptomatic women, five histologically well differentiated or partially differentiated endometrial cancers were diagnosed and one of these patients

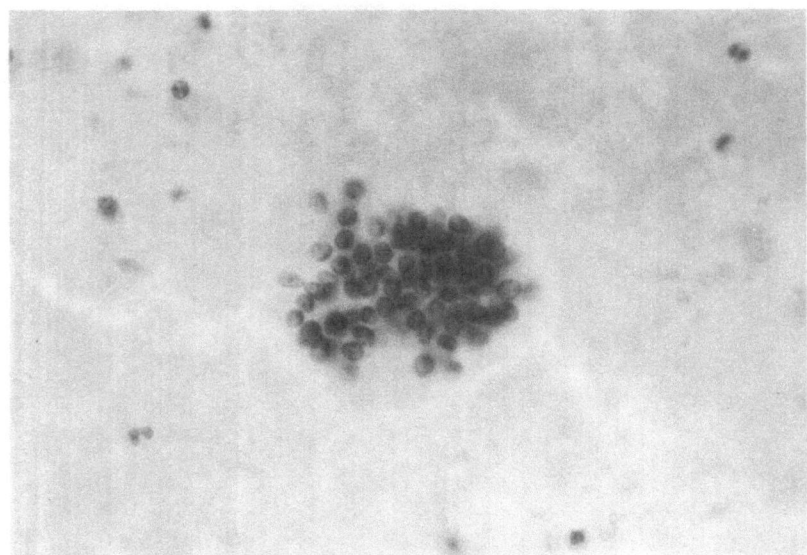

Figure 2   Benign endometrial gland cells. High power. Filter preparation

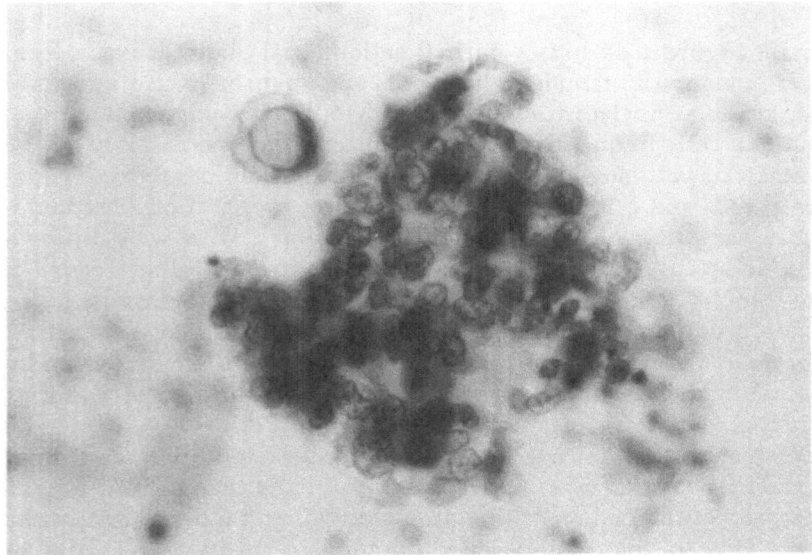

Figure 3   Adenocarcinoma of endometrium cells. High power. Filter preparation

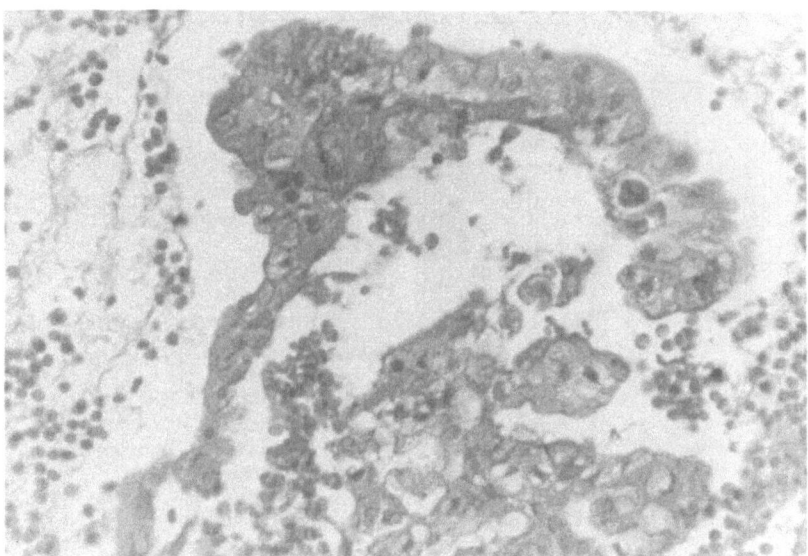

Figure 4 Adenocarcinoma of endometrium histology. High power. Cell block preparation

had been negative for cancer at the time of surgical curettage of the uterine cavity under anaesthesia less than 1 year prior to the endo-metrial irrigation. It is of special interest that the cervico-vaginal Pap smear was normal in *each* of these five patients! On the other hand, we found our cytohistological interpretation from uterine lavage to be inadequate in diagnosing non-malignant causes of uterine symptoms. Table 1 lists the clinical indications for 20 consecutive diagnostic endometrial curettages. Endometrial irrigation was carried out under anaesthesia immediately prior to surgical curettage. In this group of patients, endometrial carcinoma was accurately diagnosed in each of the three cases, but the specimens recovered were inadequate for the diagnosis of two endometrial polyps, cystic hyperplasia and adeno-matous hyperplasia[3]. This has been our overall experience. We know of no endometrial carcinoma in our series which has been missed on specimens from adequate endometrial lavage of asymptomatic or mildly symptomatic women. Many of these women have since come to surgical curettage, and some to hysterectomy, and most have been followed for over a year since the initial endometrial irrigation. Lavage

Table 1 Histological diagnosis from endometrial irrigation of 20 consecutive patients compared with curettage

Indication	Irrigation	Curetting
PMB*	adenoca.	adenoca.
PMB	mucus only	fragment em. polyp
PMB	inactive em.	atypical hyperplasia
Pap III	prolif. em.	prolif. em.—focal CGH‡
PMB	adenoca.	adenoca.
PMB	insufficient	cystic atrophy
PMB	endometritis	endometritis
Pap III	menstrual em.	menstrual em.
DUB†	prolif. em.	prolif. em.
Cervicitis	frag. benign em.	inactive em.
PMB	insufficient	prolif. em.
PMB	atrophic em.	atrophic em.
DUB	prolif. em.	prolif. em.
Pap IV	prolif. em.	prolif. em.
Pap III	benign em.	secret. em.
Dysmenorrhea	menst. em.	menst. em.
DUB	secret. em.	secret. em.
PMB	insufficient	atypical hyperplasia
PMB	adenoca.	adenoca.
PMB	insufficient	em. polyp

* PMB: post-menopausal bleeding
† DUB: dysfunctional uterine bleeding
‡ CGH: cystic glandular hyperplasia

carried out in our clinic on one patient who presented with heavy active post-menopausal uterine bleeding was deemed unsatisfactory for cytohistological examination because of excessive blood, and a cervico-vaginal Pap smear was reported to be normal. Suction curettage of the endometrial cavity under anaesthesia prior to sharp surgical curettage recovered abundant partially differentiated adenocarcinoma. Our limited experience to date with the negative pressure aspiration curette indicates that we are able to recover tissue which is excellent for histological study of both benign and neoplastic endometrium, but of course, the material is not suitable for cytological examination. These techniques are undergoing further study.

Ninety per cent of the specimens obtained by endometrial irrigation from 177 asymptomatic peri-menopausal and post-menopausal women were felt to be satisfactory for histological diagnosis. Gross tissue fragments were recovered in 105/177 (60%) of these irrigations, and the cell block preparation proved adequate for histological interpretation in 103/177 (58%). Furthermore, filter preparations from 168/177 of the irrigants were deemed adequate for cytological examination. Thus, only 4/177 (2.26%) of the specimens were inadequate to render an interpretation based on either histology, cytology or both. (Table 2).

Table 2 Adequacy of material from endometrial irrigations for cytohistology diagnosis of atypia

Successful irrigation	Cytologically adequate specimens	Histologically adequate specimens		Specimens inadequate for both cytological & histological diagnosis
		Tissue fragments	Cell block preps.	
(Successful/ no. attempted)	(No. adequate/ no. spec.)	(No. adequate/ no. spec.)	(No. adequate/ no. spec.)	(Inadequate/no. spec.)
177/201 (88%)	168/177 (95%)	105/177 (60%)	103/177 (58%)	4/177 (2.26%)

Abnormal cervico-vaginal Pap smears were obtained from 7 of 177 asymptomatic women over 40 years of age and from 13 of 40 mildly symptomatic women in whom endometrial irrigation was carried out. Endometrial irrigations were benign in four patients with inflammatory changes on cervico-vaginal Pap smears, and these patients have had no evidence of neoplastic disease on follow-up. Seven of the

Table 3 Evaluation of peri-menopausal and post-menopausal women with endometrial cells on cervical-vaginal smears

Age (years)	Menopausal status	Exogenous estrogens	Endometrial cells		Follow-up	
			Cervical smears	Endometrial irrigation	Surgical curettage	Cervical smears
54	pre	yes	normal	normal	CGH†	—
58	post	no	normal	normal	—	negative
50	pre	yes	normal	normal	—	negative
53	pre	yes	normal	normal	CGH† FAH‡	—
51	post	yes	normal	normal	—	negative
46	post	n.r.*	atypical	normal	inactive endomet.	—
54	post	yes	atypical	normal	CGH FAH	—

* n.r.: not reported
† CGH: cystic glandular hyperplasia
‡ FAH: focal adenomatous hyperplasia

patients had endometrial cells in the cervico-vaginal Pap smears, and two of these patients were interpreted as showing atypical endometrial cells in another laboratory (Table 3). We found benign cytohistology in the endometrial irrigations from each of these seven patients. Both of the patients in whom atypical endometrial cells were diagnosed in cervico-vaginal Pap smears underwent surgical uterine curettage. Benign 'inactive' endometrium was found in one patient and cystic glandular hyperplasia with focal adenomatous hyperplasia was found in the other. Endometrial irrigation recovered benign cells and tissue from each of the five women who were found to have normal endometrial cells on their cervico-vaginal Pap smears. Subsequently, three of these women have been followed with normal smears; however, benign cystic glandular hyperplasia of the endometrium was found on surgical curettage of two other patients with normal endometrial cells on the cervico-vaginal cytology, and one of these patients had focal adenomatous hyperplasia. Nine patients with abnormal squamous cells on cervico-vaginal smears were found to have cervical intraepithelial neoplasms. Each of these women had normal cytohistology on endometrial irrigation, and one of the irrigations recovered atypical squamous cells from the cervix as well.

Three of the six patients diagnosed as having endometrial carcinoma were receiving exogenous estrogens, but this may simply reflect the ratio of popular usage of these drugs in our locality. Twenty-two asymptomatic women and seven mildly symptomatic women were also known to be taking exogenous estrogens at the time of endometrial irrigation. Insufficient material for diagnosis was recovered from one symptomatic patient, while the irrigations from all of the asymptomatic patients were considered adequate for diagnosis. A tissue diagnosis was possible on 21/29 (73%) of the patients receiving estrogens, and cytological diagnosis was rendered on all but three of these endometrial irrigations. Secretory endometrium was found in two of the twelve asymptomatic patients on estrogens for whom a tissue diagnosis could be given. Slight endometrial cellular atypia was found on two uterine irrigations from women receiving estrogens, but each showed proliferative endometrium on curettage. One of these patients was asymptomatic and the other had mild metrorrhagia. Although all of the other patients receiving exogenous estrogens had normal endometrial cytology and histology, endometrial cells were found in the cervico-vaginal smears of five of these patients and uterine curettage showed endometrial hyperplasia in each of the three patients on whom it was carried out.

Patient–Physician Acceptance

The feasibility of the irrigation technique for endometrial screening of unanaesthetized patients undergoing routine out-patient examination was studied by analysis of 201 consecutive attempted irrigations on asymptomatic women between 40 and 74 years of age. Forty per cent of these patients were post-menopausal.

Introduction of the irrigator into the uterine cavity and lavage was easy or only slightly difficult in 162/201 (81%) of the patients (Table 4). Introduction and irrigation could not be accomplished in 24

Table 4 Introduction of endometrial irrigation in asymptomatic women over 40 years of age

Introduction		No. of patients		
Easy	112	(55.7%)	162	(80.6%)
Slightly difficult	50	(24.9%)		
Very difficult	15	(7.5%)	39	(19.4%)
Not accomplished	24	(11.9%)		

Table 5 Reasons for failures in 201 attempted endometrial irrigations on asymptomatic women over 40 years of age

Cervical stenosis	13
Cervical fibroid	1
Unable to insert tip	3
Small senile vagina	1
Severe discomfort	2
Inadequate suction	2
Not recorded	2
TOTAL	24

patients (12%). Thus endometrial irrigations were successful in 88% of the asymptomatic patients. The reason for the failures (Table 5) were cervical stenosis or cervical fibroid which prevented passage of the uterine sound in 14 patients. In three other patients the irrigator tip could not be passed, although the cervix could be sounded. Small senile vagina and severe discomfort led to abandoning the procedure in three patients. Although the irrigator could be passed into two other patients, suction was inadequate for lavage.

Slight or no discomfort was reported in 141/201 (74%) of the patients, and severe discomfort was expressed by only 9 (5%) of the

Table 6   Subjective evaluation of discomfort by asymptomatic women during attempted endometrial irrigation

Degree of discomfort	No. of women reporting			
None	45	(24%)	141	(74%)
Slight	96	(51%)		
Moderate	40	(21%)	49	(26%)
Severe	9	(5%)		

patients in whom uterine irrigation was attempted (Table 6). Discomfort was least and introduction was accomplished with greatest ease in multiparous patients. Discomfort tended to be greater and introduction was more difficult in post-menopausal patients, but this was more directly correlated with advancing age than with menopausal status. Those patients in whom introduction was most difficult or not accomplished expressed the most discomfort. Four of the 13 patients with cervical stenosis expressed severe discomfort when cervical sounding was attempted; albeit seven of the patients had no discomfort and two expressed only slight discomfort. Patients with cervical stenosis were both pre-menopausal and post-menopausal and ranged from 43 to 73 years of age; although most were in their fifth decade. There was no correlation of cervical stenosis with nulliparity or low parity in this study. Only two patients with cervical stenosis were known to be receiving exogenous estrogens at the time of the attempted endometrial irrigation.

Although 12.5% of the women screened complained of transient pelvic cramping following endometrial irrigation, there were no other untoward effects. Two patients felt 'lightheaded', but none experienced syncope.

SUMMARY AND CONCLUSIONS

Patients have well accepted and tolerated the endometrial irrigation technique without anaesthesia in these out-patient studies. Inability to sound a stenotic cervix was the most frequent reason for failure to accomplish endometrial irrigation. Acceptance of endometrial screening from mid-life onward might prevent this problem. This technique recovered tissue adequate for histological diagnosis of malignancy in the majority of cases and also produced material satisfactory for cytological diagnosis of atypia, a feature which enhances the value of this

Table 7 Profile of 115 patients with adenocarcinoma of the uterine corpus (New Britain General Hospital 1971–1975)

Age range (years)			Menopausal status		Weight > 150 lb	Blood sugar > 120 mg%	Exogenous thyroid	Asymptomatic with abnormal cervical smear
<40*	40–49	>50	pre	post				
3(2.6%)†	10(8.7%)	102(88.7%)	20(17.4%)	95(82.6%)	48(41.8%)	42(36.2%)	8(7%)	9(6%)

*Youngest patient was 26 years of age
† Number of patients (percentage of total)

device for the detection of small, occult endometrial cancers. In our hands, this method was inadequate for the diagnosis of endometrial hyperplasia, but Ng et al.[4, 5], have demonstrated that there is increasing exfoliation of atypical endometrial cells and cell clumps with increasing severity of endometrial pathology and dedifferentiation of adenocarcinoma.

In a review of 115 patients with endometrial carcinoma who were treated at the New Britain General Hospital between 1971 and 1975 (Table 7) only 9 were diagnosed by abnormal findings on routine cervico-vaginal Pap smear[6]. While we believe that abnormal peri-menopausal and post-menopausal bleeding demands evaluation by surgical curettage, endometrial irrigation provides us with an opportunity to obtain material adequate for histological and cytological study in the screening of asymptomatic patients at risk of developing endometrial cancer. The proven and potential risk factors for developing endometrial cancer have been discussed in detail[7, 8], and a summary is presented in Table 8. At this time we have no idea nor could we predict the impact which screening asymptomatic patients will have upon the incidence of diagnosis or cure rate of patients who are

Table 8 Candidates for endometrial screening

Family history of endometrial cancer
Previous neoplasms
   gynaecological
   rectum and colon
   breast
Delayed menopause
Endometrial hyperplasia
Stein–Leventhal syndrome
Secondary amenorrhea and infertility
High estrogen index
Exogenous estrogens
   steroidal
   non-steroidal
Obesity
Diabetes mellitus
Hypothyroidism
Exogenous thyroid
Hypertension
Oral contraceptives (?)
   sequential estrogen–progesterone
   combined estrogen–progesterone
All women over 40 years of age (?)

found to have endometrial cancer. Furthermore, as was true during the early experience with cervico-vaginal Pap smear in the detection of epidermoid carcinoma of the cervix, we have no data which would allow us to recommend the interval at which screening of asymptomatic patients should be repeated.

The negative pressure endometrial irrigation technique has been highly acceptable and accurate in our hands for the detection of endometrial carcinoma, and these findings confirm the experience of other investigators[2, 8].

Acknowledgment

We thank S. J. McLelland and A. Spitzer for their able technical assistance.

References

1. Gravlee, L. C. (1969). Jet-irrigation method for the diagnosis of endometrial carcinoma. Its principle and accuracy. *Obstet. Gynecol.*, **34**, 168
2. Casey, M. J. and Madden, T. J. (1976). Endometrial screening of asymptomatic women by irrigation technique in the private gynecology office. *J. Am. Geriatr. Soc.* (in press)
3. Casey, M. J., Kiertisak, P. and Madden, T. J. (1972). Unpublished data
4. Ng, A. B. P., Reagan, J. W., Hawliczek, C. T. and Wentz, B. W. (1974). Significance of endometrial cells in the detection of endometrial carcinoma and its precursors. *Acta Cytol.*, **18**, 356
5. Ng, A. B. P. (1974). Cellular detection of endometrial carcinoma and its precursors. *Gynecol. Oncol.*, **2**, 162
6. Kennedy, A. W., Casey, M. J. and McLucas, E. (1976). Unpublished data
7. MacMahon, B. (1974). Risk factors for endometrial cancer. *Gynecol. Oncol.*, **2**, 122
8. Casey, M. J. (1976) Estrogens, Menopause and Cancer, address to the Section on Obstetrics and Gynecology, the 184th Annual Meeting of the Connecticut State Medical Society, Hartford, April 29

24

Estrogens, Progestagens and Endometrial Cancer

R. D. Gambrell, Jr.

Wilford Hall USAF Medical Center, Lackland, Texas, USA

INTRODUCTION

Recent studies seem to implicate estrogen therapy for post-menopausal women as a possible cause of endometrial carcinoma[1-3]. Even the sequential oral contraceptives have been suggested as a possible causative agent for cancer of the endometrium in young women[4-6]. Publicity of these reports by the news media have created fears for our patients and a dilemma for the gynaecologist.

The incidence of endometrial malignancy among estrogen-treated women at Wilford Hall USAF Medical Center is apparently not as high as the 4.5–7.6 increased risk recently reported[2,3]. An attempt has been made to find this incidence and see what factors are involved in the management of our patients that lowers the anticipated risk of cancer. The role of hormones, endogenous and exogenous estrogens as well as natural and synthetic progestagens, in the production or prevention of endometrial hyperplasia and neoplasia, will be reviewed.

CLINIC POPULATION AND METHODS

There were 78 660 outpatient visits to the Obstetrics–Gynecology clinic during 1975. Unknown is the exact number of post-menopausal

The opinions expressed herein are those of the author and are not to be construed as official or reflecting the views of the Department of Defense or the United States Air Force.

women treated with estrogens. However, since there were 1 212 900 estrogen tablets dispensed from the pharmacy, and most patients take the hormones for 25 days each month (300 tablets per year), it can be calculated that there were approximately 4000 post-menopausal women receiving estrogen replacement therapy. A prospective study, started early in 1976, indicates that 42% of these women have had a previous hysterectomy, leaving 2300 patients with an intact uterus and at risk for endometrial cancer. The first month of the study further indicates that 82% of our post-menopausal women are treated with estrogens and of this group, 46% with an intact uterus take estrogens only while 54% also receive a progestagen along with the estrogen. Assuming that the first month of the study and the 393 women surveyed are representative of our clinic population, reasonable estimates of incidences can then be calculated.

RESULTS

During 1975 there were approximately 4000 post-menopausal women that received estrogen replacement therapy, 2760 taking estrogens only while 1240 had also been given a progestagen along with the estrogen (Table 1). There were 2300 women with an intact uterus and

Table 1   Adenocarcinoma of endometrium at Wilford Hall USAF Medical Center during 1975

	Estrogen users	Estrogen–progestogen users	Untreated	Total
Post-menopausal women	2760*	1240*	880*	4880*
Post hysterectomy	1700*	—	370*	2070*
Intact uterus	1060*	1240*	510*	2810*
Endometrial cancers	5	1	1	7
Cancer incidence	1:212	1:1240	1:510	1:400

* Estimated from available information

at risk for endometrial cancer. Adenocarcinoma of the endometrium was diagnosed in seven patients and six of these women had received estrogen therapy. Estrogens only was the therapy in five for an incidence of endometrial cancer in this group of one per 212 women (4.7:1000). There was one endometrial malignancy in a patient

receiving a progestagen along with the estrogen for an incidence in
this group of one per 1240 women (0.8:1000). There were approximately 510 untreated post-menopausal women with an intact uterus
in our clinic and one adenocarcinoma of the endometrium was
detected for an incidence in this group of one per 510 women
(2.0:1000).

There does not seem to be a relationship of the type and dosage of
estrogen to adenocarcinoma of the endometrium. Ethinyl estradiol
0.02 mg was the estrogen taken by approximately 400 patients without
prior hysterectomy and there was one endometrial cancer in this group
(Table 2). Conjugated estrogens 0.625 mg had been prescribed for 430

Table 2   Type and dosage of estrogen in patients with endometrial cancer

	Dosage	Patients	Cancers	Incidence
Ethinyl estradiol	0.02 mg	400*	1	1:400
Conjugated estrogens	0.625 mg	430*	2	1:215
Conjugated estrogens	1.25 mg	1470*	3	1:490
None		510*	1	1:510

* Estimated from available information

women with a uterus and two cancers were detected. The lowest
incidence of endometrial malignancy was in the group of 1470
patients that had received conjugated estrogens 1.25 mg.

The clinical characteristics of the seven patients with adenocarcinoma of the endometrium are listed in Table 3. Five were in the sixth
decade of life with one under age 50 and another age 66. Four were of
low parity, para one or less. One patient was markedly obese and three
others were moderately overweight. Significant hypertension occurred
only in one but four others had borderline elevated blood pressures.

Table 3   Clinical characteristics: adenocarcinoma of endometrium

Patient	Age	Para	Weight	BP
VDMcL	56	0000	169 lb	144/90
MRH	53	3003	150 lb	140/80
JAC	55	1001	—	110/76
RM	52	2012	130 lb	150/80
EGR	46	1011	123 lb	104/70
HBA	58	0000	160 lb	152/86
MLF	66	3003	198 lb	180/100

Table 4 Hormonal therapy of patients with adenocarcinoma of endometrium

Patient	Estrogen therapy	Method	Duration	Progestogen
VDMcL	Ethinyl estradiol 0.02 mg	1st–25th/mo	2½ yrs	None
MRH	Conjugated estrogens 0.625 mg	1st–25th/mo	7 yrs	None
JAC	Conjugated estrogens 0.625 mg	1st–25th/mo	3 yrs	None
RM	Conjugated estrogens 1.25 mg	Daily	10 yrs	None
EGR	Conjugated estrogens 1.25 mg	1st–25th/mo	3 yrs	None
HBA	Conjugated estrogens 1.25 mg	1st–25th/mo	7 yrs	Medroxyprogesterone 10 mg 21st–25th/mo
MLF	None	—	—	None

Table 5 Endometrial cancers referred to Wilford Hall USAF Medical Center during 1975

Therapy	Number
Estrogen	10
No hormones	11
Oracon	1
Total cases	22

Table 6 Estrogen therapy and endometrial malignancy

Year	Estrogen users	Total cancers
1972	Unknown	6
1973	Unknown	5
1974	3200*	7
1975	4000*	7

* Estimated from available information

Hormonal therapy is listed in Table 4. Five of the six patients receiving estrogens were on cyclic therapy and had been taking hormones from 2½ to 7 years. One patient had been receiving continuous daily estrogens for 10 years. Only one was also taking a progestagen, medroxyprogesterone, 10 mg/day from the 21st–25th of the month for the previous 2 years.

In addition to the seven endometrial cancers from our clinic population, 22 cases were diagnosed elsewhere and referred to Wilford Hall USAF Medical Center for treatment in 1975 (Table 5). Eleven

(50%) of these had received no hormones while ten were taking estrogens and one was receiving Oracon for birth control. None of the ten women taking estrogens had also been given a progestagen. No apparent increase in the frequency of adenocarcinoma of the endometrium has been noticed in our clinic population in recent years. There were six endometrial cancers in 1972 as compared to seven cases in 1975 (Table 6).

Endometrial hyperplasia had been previously diagnosed in three of

Table 7   Endometrial cancer with previous hyperplasia of endometrium

Patient	Date	Pathology
VDMcL	March 1975	Benign endometrial hyperplasia
	November 1975	Adenocarcinoma of endometrium
HBA	May 1973	Focal adenomatous hyperplasia
	July 1975	Adenocarcinoma of endometrium
JAC	September 1967	Cystic glandular hyperplasia
	March 1975	Adenocarcinoma of endometrium

Table 8   Effects of 19-nor steroid progestagens on endometrial hyperplasia

Pathology before therapy	Number	Endometrium after therapy	Number
Benign hyperplasia	42	Proliferative	30
Cystic hyperplasia	9	Secretory	13
Adenomatous hyperplasia	5	Atrophic	11
Atypical adenomatous		Dyssynchronous maturation	5
hyperplasia	4	Benign hyperplasia	1
Total patients	60	Total patients	60

our seven patients from 8 months to 8 years before the detection of cancer (Table 7). During the past 4 years, 60 patients with varying degrees of endometrial hyperplasia have been treated with a synthetic 19-nor steroid progestagen. The majority were peri-menopausal women and not receiving any hormonal therapy. The pathology before progestogen therapy and histology of the endometrium after treatment are listed in Table 8. Following 3 months of treatment with either norethindrone acetate or norgestrelethinyl estradiol, repeat curettage indicated that the hyperplasia had reverted to normal endometrium in 59 of the 60 cases. In the one patient where the hyperplasia persisted, a hysterectomy was performed; however, no hyperplasia was found in the surgical specimen.

The progestagen chosen to treat dysfunctional uterine bleeding after office curettage, was as follows. To arrest acute bleeding, Ovral is administered, three tablets the first day and two tablets for 9 days, followed by one tablet daily, 21 out of 28 days for two additional cycles. To treat chronic bleeding, after curettage, norethindrone acetate 5 mg daily, is prescribed from the 19th to the 25th of either the cycle or the month. If the patient was already taking an estrogen, it was continued cyclicly. There were 29 patients with hyperplasia treated with Ovral and 31 were given norethindrone acetate.

COMMENT

There are several recent retrospective studies that seem to implicate estrogen therapy for post-menopausal women as a possible cause of endometrial carcinoma[1-3]. The incidence of endometrial malignancy for all ages in the United States is 21 per 100 000 women[7]. Quint was the first to report in 1975 the changing incidence of endometrial cancer[1]. He divided his study into two periods and in the early period, few post-menopausal women received estrogen therapy. In the later period with increased estrogen usage, the risk of endometrial cancer increased 1.8-fold. In a second study of 317 patients with adeno-carcinoma of the endometrium, the matched controls were patients with other gynaecological malignancies and the risk of endometrial cancer was 4.5 times greater among women exposed to estrogen therapy[2]. In another study of 94 patients with carcinoma of the endo-metrium, there were two matched controls for each patient, who were apparently healthy, and the estimated risk ratio was 7.6 for estrogen treated women[3].

To put these figures in proper perspective, there is a 3 to 9-fold increased risk for endometrial cancer in association with obesity alone[8]. There is a 17-fold increased risk of death from lung cancer in those who smoke 20 cigarettes per day[9]. Other studies have shown that women treated with estrogen have a reduction in both mortality and total cancer incidence[10]. In one such report, where all the women had undergone hysterectomy, the expected mortality was reduced by 58%[11] in post-menopausal women receiving estrogen therapy. The lowest mortality for all gynaecological malignancies, regardless of staging, is endometrial cancer. The probability that untreated post-menopausal women with an intact uterus will develop carcinoma of the endometrium is 1:1000 per year[10]. With estrogen users, according to the recent studies, it is increased to 1.8–7.6:1000 women per year.

Our data for a single year indicate that the incidence of endometrial cancer among estrogen users is 2.6:1000, including those also taking a progestagen. In addition, of the 22 cases of adenocarcinoma of the endometrium referred to Wilford Hall USAF Medical Center for treatment, 50% had received no estrogens.

Prophylactic hysterectomy prior to estrogen therapy would prevent this increased risk; however, 992 of 1000 women would have needless surgery. The alternative to hysterectomy prior to estrogen replacement therapy may be to add progestagens. In one of the studies about the changing pattern in endometrial carcinoma, none of the 291 women had been treated with a progestagen, although the author stated that it would be his future practice[1]. In the two other studies[2,3], progestagens were not mentioned.

The incidence of endometrial cancer during 1975 among all estrogen users in our clinic was 2.6:1000 women. In the patients receiving only an estrogen, the incidence of malignancy was 4.7:1000, which is in the range of the other retrospective studies[2,3]. However, in our patients that also received a progestagen with the estrogen, only one cancer was detected for an incidence of 0.8:1000. This is lower than the spontaneous occurrence of adenocarcinoma of the endometrium in untreated post-menopausal women[10].

Oral contraceptive therapy has been implicated in 28 reported cases of endometrial cancer with 24 of the patients under the age of 40[4–6]. The sequential pill, principally Oracon, was used by 20, combined pills by seven, and in one patient, the pill was unknown. In the largest study, seven of 21 patients had discontinued oral contraceptives for 8 months to 6 years before the diagnosis of endometrial carcinoma[6]. Contrary to the opinion of the authors, these patients should receive separate consideration since progestagens can only be effective in preventing hyperplasia and neoplasia while they are being administered.

Other factors need to be considered. The 100 μg of ethinyl estradiol in Oracon is a much higher dosage than the 20 μg of this estrogen or 0.625–1.25 mg of conjugated estrogens usually given post-menopausal women. The progestagen in Oracon is dimethisterone, which is a C-19 compound and not a 19-nor steroid like all the other progestagens in the birth control pills. Furthermore, the 5 days of dimethisterone may not be sufficient, for this somewhat weak progestagen, to produce complete endometrial shedding, especially in view of the relatively high dosage of ethinyl estradiol in this birth control pill. Epidemiological studies will probably indicate a decreased incidence of carcinoma of the endometrium with combined pills, and that sequential pills may not be as protective.

It has long been recognized that there are predisposing factors to the development of endometrial carcinoma. These include: obesity, hypertension, diabetes, and infertility. In one series of 229 cases of adenocarcinoma of the endometrium from the United States, 66.2% were of low parity, 71.4% had hypertension, obesity was found in 64%, and diabetes was present in 28%[12]. In another study of 150 cases from Italy[13], nulliparity, diabetes and obesity were frequent findings but hypertension was not a predisposing factor. In this report, pregnancy (even those ending in abortion) seemed to limit future endometrial malignancy. The patient profile for endometrial cancer is the single or nulliparous woman, particularly in the presence of diabetes, obesity, and continued natural menses after age 50[14].

Extensive work done by MacDonald and his group[15-17] have indicated the changes in hormone production after menopause that may lead to endometrial neoplasia. To summarize their very important data, endogenous estrogens may rise in post-menopausal women either due to increased production rate of androstenedione or a greater peripheral conversion of this prehormone to estrone. Furthermore, it has been reported that in obese women there is a greater percentage conversion of androstenedione to estrone. Women produce very little progesterone after the menopause.

For over a decade it has been my policy to add a progestagen to the estrogen therapy of all post-menopausal women with an intact uterus[18]. Time has not altered my convictions, only strengthened them. To be sure, women look forward to that time in life when they are through with menstrual periods and are very reluctant to have them reinstituted. However, with a careful explanation, a return of menses can be accepted. Not all patients receiving estrogen replacement therapy must have withdrawal bleeding. If the estrogen dosage given to relieve menopausal symptoms is sufficient to induce proliferation of the endometrium, as evidenced by withdrawal menses from a progestagen, then this progestagen should be continued cyclicly as long as withdrawal bleeding follows. If withdrawal bleeding does not take place during 3 months of such therapy, it is presumed safe to discontinue the progestagen.

Unopposed estrogens apparently have a role in the aetiology of

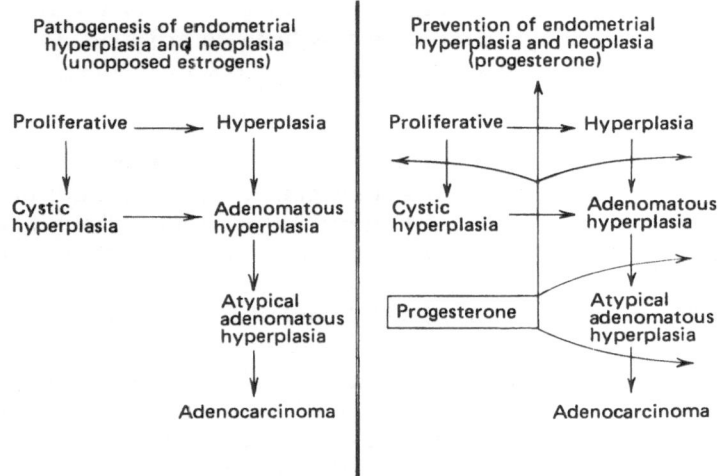

Figure 1 Schematic representation of how estrogen unopposed by progesterone may lead to progressive hyperplastic changes. By producing more complete endometrial shedding, progesterone may interrupt progressive hyperplastic changes resulting from unopposed estrogens

endometrial hyperplasia and neoplasia through incomplete shedding of the endometrium (Figure 1). Progesterone not only produces a more complete sloughing of the endometrium, but also converts all degrees of hyperplasia to secretory endometrium in nearly all cases. Evidence for the importance of unopposed estrogens may be demonstrated in many ways. Nulliparity, infertility, and anovulation are primary predisposing factors to endometrial carcinoma[1, 13, 14]. Secretory endometrium is present in only 1.0–1.9% of patients with post-menopausal bleeding[19, 20], and almost never found concomitantly with adenocarcinoma of the endometrium. Progestagens are standard palliative therapy for metastatic endometrial cancer[21]. They can also reverse hyperplasia to normal endometrium.

In our treatment of endometrial hyperplasia, 29 patients with varying degrees, including severe atypical adenomatous hyperplasia, were given norgestrel-ethinyl estradiol. Another 31 were treated with norethindrone acetate. The endometrium reverted to normal in 59 of the 60 cases.

Progestagens that are 19-nor testosterone derivatives, such as norethindrone and norgestrel, seem to be superior to other progestagens for preventing and treating endometrial hyperplasia. In a study of 53 post-menopausal patients treated for up to 16 years with continuous estrogens with or without progestagen therapy, 12 (22.6%) developed cystic or adenomatous hyperplasia[22]. There were no endometrial cancers in this series. Medroxyprogesterone, dydrogesterone, and chlormadinone, all C-21 compounds, were the progestagens in seven of the eight receiving this type of combined therapy. Only one patient treated with a 19-nor steroid progestagen, methylestrenolone, developed cystic hyperplasia while undergoing therapy. The remaining four patients had been given continuous estrogens only. Treatment of patients with adenomatous hyperplasia by lynestrenol, also a 19-nor steroid progestagen, reversed the lesions in all four. In another report of 25 patients treated with continuous daily ethinyl estradiol of graduated dosage up to 125 μg/day, which is a very high dosage, 94% developed hyperplasia of the endometrium[23]. When medroxyprogesterone 10 mg was added to the last 7 days of estrogen therapy, 6% still developed hyperplasia. In our only patient that developed adenocarcinoma during combined estrogen–progestagen therapy, medroxyprogesterone was the progestagen given for only 5 days each month, therapy probably too short for adequate sloughing.

Hyperplasia of the endometrium, regardless of degree, is almost invariably reversed with progestagen therapy. Patients with any degree of hyperplasia of the endometrium must have a repeat curettage after three months of therapy. Should the hyperplasia persist, a hysterectomy is performed. Withdrawal bleeding from 19-nor steroid progestagens almost invariably occurs 2–3 days after the last tablet and rarely lasts for more than 3–5 days. Any variation from this planned withdrawal bleeding requires a repeat office curettage. However, in the few instances where this has been necessary, the tissue was normal: proliferative, secretory, or dyssynchronous maturation[24].

Estrogen replacement therapy is given to a woman with an intact uterus only with a progestagen added for at least 3 months trial. To date, not a single patient has developed hyperplasia or neoplasia while undergoing such therapy when a 19-nor steroid progestagen was used.

CONCLUSIONS

1. There is probably some increased risk of endometrial cancer from estrogen therapy for menopause.

2. This risk may not be as great with cyclic estrogens.

3. Progestagens, particularly 19-nor steroids, may minimise and possibly eliminate, this increased risk.

References

1. Quint, B. C. (1975). Changing patterns in endometrial adenocarcinoma. *Am. J. Obstet. Gynecol.*, **122**, 498
2. Smith, D. C., Prentice, R., Thompson, D. J. and Herrman, W. L. (1975). Association of exogenous estrogen and endometrial carcinoma. *N. Engl. J. Med.*, **293**, 1164
3. Ziel, H. K. and Finkle, W. D. (1975). Increased risk of endometrial carcinoma among users of conjugated estrogens. *N. Engl. J. Med.*, **293**, 1167
4. Kelly, H. W., Miles, P. A., Buster, J. E. and Scragg, W. H. (1976). Adenocarcinoma of the endometrium in women taking sequential oral contraceptives. *Obstet. Gynecol.*, **47**, 200
5. Lyon, F. A. (1975). The development of adenocarcinoma of the endometrium in young women receiving long-term sequential oral contraceptives. Report of four cases. *Am. J. Obstet. Gynecol.*, **123**, 299
6. Silverberg, S. G. and Makowski, E. L. (1975). Endometrial carcinoma in young women taking oral contraceptive agents. *Obstet. Gynecol.*, **46**, 503
7. Levin, D. L., Devessa, S. S., Godwin, J. D. II and Silverman, D. T. (1974). *Cancer Rates and Risks*, p. 13. (Washington: Department of Health, Education, and Welfare)
8. Gusberg, S. B. (1975). A strategy for the control of endometrial cancer. *Proc. R. Soc. Med.*, **68**, 163
9. Ryan, K. J. (1975). Cancer risk and estrogen use in the menopause. *N. Engl. J. Med.*, **293**, 1199
10. Weiss, N. S. (1975). Risks and benefit of estrogen use. *N. Engl. J. Med.*, **293**, 1200
11. Burch, J. C., Byrd, B. F. Jr and Vaughn, W. K. (1974). The effects of long-term estrogen on hysterectomized women. *Am. J. Obstet. Gynecol.*, **118**, 778
12. Mickal, A. and Torres, J. (1974). Adenocarcinoma of endometrium. In *The Menopausal Syndrome*, R. B. Greenblatt, V. B. Mahesh and P. G. McDonough (eds.), pp. 139–142. (New York: Medcom, Inc.)
13. Centaro, A., Ceci, G., De Laurentis, G. and De Salvia, D. (1974). Epidemiologic studies of post-menopausal endometrial adenocarcinoma. In *The Menopausal Syndrome*, R. B. Greenblatt, V. B. Mahesh and P. G. McDonough (eds.), pp. 133–138. (New York: Medcom, Inc.)
14. Kistner, R. W., Krantz, K. E., Lebherz, T. B. *et al.* (1973). Endometrial cancer: Rising incidence, detection, and treatment. *J. Reprod. Med.*, **10**, 53
15. Hemsell, D. L., Siiteri, P. K. and MacDonald, P. C. (1972). Estrogen derived from plasma androstenedione. Presentation to the *Armed Forces District Meeting of the American College of Obstetricians and Gynecologists*, Seattle, October, 1972.
16. Hemsell, D. L., Siiteri, P. K., MacDonald, P. C. *et al.* (1974). Plasma precursors of estrogen. II. Correlation of the extent of conversion of plasma androstenedione to estrone with age. *J. Clin. Endocrinol. Metab.*, **38**, 467
17. MacDonald, P. C. and Siiteri, P. K. (1974). The relationship between the extraglandular production of estrone and the occurrence of endometrial neoplasia. *Gynecol. Oncol.*, **2**, 259

18. Gambrell, R. D. Jr. (1974). Perimenopausal and postmenopausal bleeding: Mechanisms, pathology, management with progestational agents. In *The Menopausal Syndrome*, R. B. Greenblatt, V. B. Mahesh and P. G. McDonough (eds.), pp. 147-156. (New York: Medcom, Inc.)

19. Gambrell, R. D. Jr. (1974). Postmenopausal bleeding. *J. Am. Geriat. Soc.*, **22**, 337

20. Procopé, B-J. (1971). Aetiology of postmenopausal bleeding. *Acta Obstet. Gynecol. Scand.*, **50**, 311

21. Kistner, R. W. and Griffiths, C. T. (1968). Use of progestational agents in the management of metastatic carcinoma of the endometrium. *Clin. Obstet. Gynecol.*, **11**, 439

22. Ferin, J. (1974). Effect of replacement therapy on endometrium in postmenopausal women. In *The Menopausal Syndrome*, R. B. Greenblatt, V. B. Mahesh and P. G. McDonough (eds.), pp. 143-146. (New York: Medcom, Inc.)

23. Dalla Pria S., Lebech, P. E., McEwen, D. C. *et al.* (1974). Hormone therapy of menopause: A panel. In *The Menopausal Syndrome*, R. B. Greenblatt, V. B. Mahesh and P. G. McDonough (eds.), pp. 197–221. (New York: Medcom, Inc.)

24. Gambrell, R. D. Jr. and Greenblatt, R. B. (1975). Management of dysfunctional uterine bleeding with norgestrel-ethinyl estradiol. *Curr. Med. Dialog.*, **42**, 80

25

Results of Estrogen Treatment in One Thousand Hysterectomized Women for 14 318 years

J. C. Burch, B. F. Byrd and W. K. Vaughn
Vanderbilt University, Nashville, Tennessee, USA

The end of the fertile period of life is marked by the menopause or cessation of menstruation. The post-menopause is long and often occupies one third or more of the life span. It may be accompanied by a period of mental and physical unrest which may be severe.

According to Kistner, the average age of menopause is 48. Jaszman gives 51.4 years with a standard deviation of 3.75 years. In the 5th and 6th centuries, the stated figure was 50 years with only 28% of the women surviving to that age and only 5% reaching 75. Today the lengthening of the post-menopausal period has produced a population which equals one third of the total population.

The critical period of a woman's life is the long post-reproductive phase which is characterized by severe ovarian failure with a severe or even complete lack of estrogen. This results in a general decline of every tissue in her body. Fortunately, this can be largely offset by the administration of estrogen.

The hysterectomized woman with ovarian failure offers an ideal subject to study for the general effects of estrogen replacement without the uterine effects. At the present we have accumulated 1000 cases of ovarian failure without the uterus. These patients have been on estrogen since the onset of this failure. If the ovaries were removed, estrogen was started at once, if they were conserved, estrogen was started at the time of the appearance of estrogen deficiency symptoms.

Table 1   Observed and expected incidence of all cancer, all patients

Age	Number of patient years	Expected[1]	Observed
25–29	68.250	0.030	0
30–34	298.333	0.237	0
35–39	885.667	1.224	2
40–44	1860.417	4.145	4
45–49	2753.417	8.968	3
50–54	3075.000	14.763	10
55–59	2453.917	15.442	16
60–64	1641.917	14.347	10
65–69	848.167	8.763	8
70–74	316.000	4.221	1
75–79	87.667	1.378	
80–84	24.083	0.448	2
85–89	4.833	0.100	
Unknown			7
TOTAL	14 317.652	74.066	63

Estrogen has such a proliferative effect on the entire genital tract that it naturally raises the question of its carcinogenic effect. This is what is uppermost in the minds of both patients and physicians (Table 1).

During the time of this study, 1000 hysterectomized women with ovarian failure were observed for a total period of 14 318 years. This amounts to 14.318 years per patient. During this period, 74.006

Table 2   Observed and expected deaths from all cancer, all patients

Age	Number of patient years	Expected[1]	Observed
25–29	68.250	0.008	0
30–34	298.333	0.067	0
35–39	885.667	0.478	0
40–44	1860.417	1.005	4
45–49	2753.417	4.185	3
50–54	3075.000	4.674	3
55–59	2453.917	6.896	5
60–64	1641.917	4.614	5
65–69	848.167	4.148	3
70–74	316.000	1.545	1
75–79	87.667	0.754	0
80–84	24.083	0.205	0
85–89	4.833	0.059	0
TOTAL	14 317.652	28.628	23

patients were expected to develop cancer. Actually, only 63 did develop cancer. This is only 85.128% of the expected normal. Of those patients developing cancer, 28.628 cases were expected to die (Table 2). In fact only 23 died (80.341%).

Table 3   Expected and observed breast cancer incidence, all patients

	Number of patient years	Expected [1]	Observed
TOTAL	14 317.652	23.701	33

Breast cancer was expected to develop in 23.701 cases, while in reality 33 were observed. This is 39% more than was expected (Table 3).

Table 4   Expected and observed deaths from breast cancer, all patients

	Number of patient years	Expected [1]	Observed
TOTAL	14 317.652	7.852	6

Table 5   Observed and expected deaths from heart conditions, all patients

Age	Number of patient years	Expected [1]	Observed
25–29	68.250	0.006	0
30–34	298.333	0.035	0
35–39	885.667	0.201	0
40–44	1860.417	0.422	1
45–49	2753.417	2.453	0
50–54	3075.000	2.740	4
55–59	2453.917	7.428	0
60–64	1641.917	4.970	2
65–69	848.167	8.982	2
70–74	316.000	3.346	2
75–79	87.667	3.642	0
80–84	24.083	1.000	2
85–89	4.833	0.201	0
TOTAL	14 317.652	35.427	13

Deaths from breast cancer were expected in 7.85 cases while only 6 cases were observed (Table 4). This is 76.4% of the expected. While the incidences of breast cancer was up 39%, its mortality was down

23.6%. More cancer resulting in less deaths suggests greater host resistance or less virulence.

Before giving estrogens, mammograms are advisable. The breast should be examined regularly by the patient and every 6 months by the physician. Under these circumstances the danger of cancer can be reduced.

At present there is no known evidence that coronary heart disease is prevented or delayed by estrogen. But a decrease from the expected 35.427 deaths from heart disease to 13 or 63% casts a different picture on the situation (Table 5).

Table 6   Expected and observed CVA deaths, all patients

Age	Number of patient years	Expected[1]	Observed
25–29	68.250	0.001	0
30–34	298.333	0.006	0
35–39	885.667	0.122	0
40–44	1860.417	0.257	2
45–49	2753.417	0.950	1
50–54	3075.000	1.061	1
55–59	2453.917	2.805	2
60–64	1641.917	1.877	2
65–69	848.167	3.890	0
70–74	316.000	1.449	0
75–79	87.667	1.501	0
80–84	24.083	0.412	0
85–89	4.833	0.199	0
TOTAL	14 317.652	14.530	8

Table 7   Expected and observed fracture of the wrist, all patients

	Number of patient years	Expected[1]	Observed
TOTAL	14 317.652	40.200	12

The decline in deaths from CVA of 14.530 to 8, further strengthens the belief that estrogen delays the ageing of arteries (Table 6).

The decrease from an expected 40.200 in fractures of the wrist to 12 is 70% decrease. This is certainly in keeping with the accepted theory that estrogens are a known inhibitor of bone resorption (Table 7).

Table 8   Expected and observed deaths from accidents, all patients

	Number of patient years	Expected[1]	Observed
TOTAL	14 317.652	3.728	5

The deaths from accidents are included only for completeness (Table 8).

Table 9   Observed and expected deaths, all patients

Age	Number of patient years	Expected[1]	Observed
25–29	68.250	0.082	0
30–34	298.333	0.477	0
35–39	885.667	2.037	0
40–44	1860.417	6.139	7
45–49	2753.417	13.492	5
50–54	3075.000	22.755	10
55–59	2453.917	26.993	10
60–64	1641.917	28.734	10
65–69	848.167	24.512	6
70–74	316.000	14.726	4
75–79	87.667	6.531	0
80–84	24.083	1.794	2
85–89	4.833	0.360	0
TOTAL	14 317.652	148.632	54

Of paramount importance, the overall death rate of the 1000 hysterectomized women observed for 14.318 years was reduced from an expected 148.632 to 54 (Table 9). This will result in an improvement in life expectancy above the US normal of about 4.14 years at age 52.

CONCLUSION

The documented results from the 1000 observed women are highly significant to the question—are they carcinogenic? The observed results strongly suggest they are not.

Seventy-four patients were expected to develop cancer while only 63 did. Of the 63 developing cancer, 29 were expected to die, while only 23 did die. Thus, the general incidence of cancer or its mortality is not increased but actually decreased. However, there was an increase of 39% in breast cancer, but the deaths from breast cancer were down from 8 to 6. All other cancers and deaths from cancer were down. In addition, the general bodily effects are shown in the decreased number of fractures of the wrist and the lowering of the death rate from heart disease and strokes.

Furthermore, the expected overall death rate was dramatically reduced.

Reference

1. Dorn, H. F. and Cutler, S. J. (1965). Morbidity from cancer in the United States. Cancer Morbidity Series, U.S. Public Health (1947/48). *Tennessee Department of Public Health: Annual Bulletin of Vital Statistics (1965)*

Section C

Free Communications :

A Comprehensive List of all the Papers
Presented at the Congress

Free Communications

(Papers marked with an asterisk are given in full in Section B)

Free Communications I **Psycho-social Aspects**

* Marcha Flint, 'Cross-cultural Factors That Affect Age of Menopause'. Department of Anthropology, Montclair State College,
  Upper Montclair, NJ 07043, USA

S. Matsumoto, 'Age at Menopause in Japanese Women and Pre-
  Menopausal Menstrual Cycles'. Department of Obstetrics and
  Gynaecology, Jichi Medical School. Address: Tsuruta-machi
  1704-31, Utsonomiya 320, Japan

* G. Vanhulle and R. Demol. 'A Double-Blind Investigation into
  the Effect of Estriol on a Number of Psychological Tests in Post-
  menopausal Women'. Dorpstraat 190, 3060 Bertem, Belgium

M. A. Weill-Hallé, 'Complaintes des Femmes au prèsde leur Médecin
  à propos de leur Ménopause'. 77 av. Paul Doumer, Paris 16e,
  France

D. G. Hertz, 'Dreaming Process and Fantasy-Life in Menopausal
  Women'. Psychiatric Clinic, Hebrew University, Hadassah Medical
  School, PO Box 499, Jerusalem, Israel

* Mitjam Furuhjelm and P. Fedor-Freybergh, 'The Influence of
  Estrogen on the Psyche in Climacteric and Post-menopausal

Women'. Sabbatsbergs Kvinnoklinik, Karolinska Institutet, Stockholm, Sweden

E. Schleyer-Saunders, 'The Menopause, a Gerontological Problem'. 56 Wimpole St., London W1M 7DF, England

Free Communications II **Gonadotrophins**

U. Larsson-Cohn, B. Kågedal and E. Johansson, 'Effects of Postmenopausal Treatment with Ethinyl Estradiol and Estradiol Valerianate on Plasma Levels of FHS, LH and Estrone'. Linköping University, Department of Obstetrics and Gynaecology, Regionsjukhuset, 581 85 Linköping, Sweden

S. Geller, 'The Clomifene–Dexamethasone Test. Its Application to the Diagnosis of Menopause in Clinical Practice'. Laboratoire d'Hormonologie, Centre d'Exploration Fonctionnelle et d'Etude de la Reproduction Humaine (CEFER), 21 rue Ed. Rostand, 13006 Marseille, France

A. Netter, 'A Hormonal Study of Pre-menopause'. Endocrino-Gynécologie, Reproduction Humaine, Hôpital Necker, 149 rue de Sèvres, Paris 15e, France

I. Mori, M. Arima, N. Takeda, S. Kono, Y. Tsuneyoshi, T. Ikeda and S. Takenaka, 'Endocrinological Studies on Ageing of the Ovary'. Department of Obstetrics and Gynaecology, Faculty of Medicine, Kagoshima University, 1208-1 Usuki-cho, Kagoshima-shi 890, Japan

K. Ichinoe, H. Yokota, Y. Mabuchi and Y. Okada, 'Offspring from Aged Animals Grafted with Young Ovaries'. Department of Obstetrics and Gynaecology, Wakayama Medical College, Wakayama, Japan

Free Communications III **Some Effects of Estrogens**

H.-P. Klotz, M. L. Delorme and C. Aussenard, 'Mode of Action of Estrogens on Bone'. Hôpital Beaujon, Service d'Endocrinologie et de Métabolisme, 100 Bd. Général Leclerc, 92110 Clichy, France

* J. Dequeker and J. Ferin, 'The Effect of Long-Term Estrogen Therapy on Bone Remodelling in Women with a Natural Menopause: Cross-sectional and Longitudinal Study'. Rheumatology

Unit, Academic Hospital, University of Louvain, Weligervel 1, 3041 Pellenberg, Belgium

B. E. C. Nordin, 'Calcium Metabolism and the Menopause'. MRC Mineral Metabolism Unit, The General Infirmary, Great George Street, Leeds LS1 3EX, England

* H. C. van Paassen, S. A. Duursma, J. M. M. Roelofs, R. Andriesse, J. v. d. Sluys Veer and M. A. H. M. Wiegerinck, 'Biochemical Parameters of Bone Metabolism in the Pre-, Peri- and Post-menopausal State', University Hospital, Utrecht, the Netherlands

M. Notelovitz, 'The Clinical and Biochemical Assessment of Estrogen-Induced Side-effects in Post-menopausal Women'. Department of Obstetrics and Gynecology, University of Florida College of Medicine, Gainesville, FL 32610, USA

J. L. Ambrus, C. M. Ambrus, M. A. Lillie and K. Niswander, 'The Effect of Estrogens and Progestins on Blood Coagulation, Fibrinolysis and the Incidence of Thromboembolism in Women of Various Ages'. State University of New York at Buffalo, 666 Elm, Buffalo, NY 14203, USA

Free Communications IV **Clinical Aspects 1**

L. Boykin, 'Iron Deficiency Anaemia in Post-menopausal Women'. Hunter College, Bellevue School of Nursing, City University of New York, 440 East 26th Street, New York, NY 10010, USA

* E. Vázquez, H. J. Casares and J. A. Sereno, 'Influence of the Nutritional Status upon the Response of Menopausal Women to Estrogen Therapy'. Sector de Endocrinología, Departamento de Ginecología y Obstetricia, Hospital Español, Ejército Nacional 613, México 5, DF

* M. J. Casey and T. J. Madden, 'Experience with Endometrial Irrigations in Menopausal Women'. Department of Obstetrics and Gynecology, University of Connecticut, School of Medicine, Farmington, CT 06032, USA

D. J. Aravantinos, P. Calfopoulos, N. Gourzis and D. Kaskarelis, 'Clinical and Histopathological Pattern During the Pre-, Peri- and Post-menopausal Period'. State and University Maternity Hospital Alexandra, 1st Department of Obstetrics and Gynecology, Queen Sophie Avenue and C Louros Street, Athens 611, Greece

* R. D. Gambrell, Jr., 'Estrogens, Progestagens and Endometrial Cancer'. Department of Obstetrics and Gynecology, Wilford Hall USAF Medical Center, Lackland AFB, TX 78236, USA

* J. C. Burch, B. F. Byrd and W. K. Vaughn, 'Results of Estrogen Treatment in One Thousand Hysterectomized Women for 14 318 Years'. Departments of Obstetrics and Gynecology, Surgery and Biostatistics, Vanderbilt University, Nashville, Tenn, USA

J. Teter, 'Changing Concepts in Estrogen Replacement Therapy'. Department of Clinical Endocrinology, Medical Academy, 02–015 Warsaw, Pl. Starynkiewicza 1/3, Poland

Free Communications V **Clinical Aspects 2**

T. Abe, N. Furuhashi, Y. Yamaya, M. Suzuki, K. Takahashi and T. Moritsuka, 'Differences between Effects of Conjugated Estrogen on Neurotics and Non-neurotic Climacteric Women Complaining of Menopausal Symptoms'. Department of Obstetrics and Gynaecology, Tohoku University School of Medicine, 1–1 Seiryo-machi, Sendai 980, Japan

T. Ikeda, T. Ueda, S. Kamatsuki, M. Arima, K. Mihara, I. Mori and N. Ogawa, 'Psychosomatic Aspects of the Effect of Conjugated Estrogens in Patients with Post-operative Ovarian Deficiency Syndrome (a Double-Blind Study)'. Department of Obstetrics and Gynaecology, School of Medicine, Kagoshima University, 1208–1 Usuki-cho, Kagoshima-shi 890, Japan

E. Nishida, K. Akasofy, Y. Tomita and K. Araki, 'Effects of Administration of Dehydroepiandrosterone on Post-menopausal Women'. Department of Gynaecology and Obstetrics, School of Medicine, Kanazawa University, Kanazawa-920, Japan

J. H. Branolte and A. M. C. M. Schellen, 'Micronized Estradiol + Estriol for Oral Estrogen Replacement Therapy of Menopausal Complaints'. Gynaecological Department, R.C. Hospital, Sittard, The Netherlands

F. P. Rhoades, 'Continuous Cyclic Hormonal Therapy'. American Geriatric Society, 272 Ashland Avenue, Detroit, Mich 48215, USA

H. Rozenbaum, 'Traitement de la Ménopause par un Miniséquentiel contenant 30 mg d'éthinyl-estradiol'. 22 rue Emeriau, Paris 15e, France

P. L. Martin, A. Burnier and M. O. Greaney, Jr, '17β-Estradiol for Oral Estrogen Replacement Therapy'. 550 Washington Street, Suite 529, San Diego, Calif 92103, USA

Free Communications VI **Clinical Aspects 3**

T. Schneider, 'Management of Peri-menopausal Bleeding with Injectable, Long-Acting Progesterone'. Louisiana State University Medical School, New Orleans, USA

B. E. C. Nordin and B. Pelc, 'The Relation Between Plasma Androstenedione and Estrone Levels and Androstenedione to Estrone Conversion in Post-menopausal Women'. MRC Mineral Metabolism Unit, The General Infirmary, Great George Street, Leeds LS1 3EX, England

* R. Punnonen and L. Rauramo, 'The Effect of Castration and Oral Estrogen Therapy on Serum Lipids'. Department of Obstetrics and Gynaecology, University of Turku, Turku, Finland

R. M. Klapper, 'Ocular Manifestations of the Menopause'. 241 Central Park West, New York, NY 10024, USA

J. E. Rodriguez-Soriano, 'Résultats de l'Evaluation des Métrorragies de la Post-Ménopause sur 16.000 Patientes'. Departmento de Ginecologia, Hospital del Sagrado Corazon, Paris 83, Barcelona, Spain

I. Bernard, 'Treatment of Troubles of the Climacteric'. 41 rue d'Aviau, 33000 Bordeaux, France

J. Mirouze, L. Monnier, J. L. Selam and J. Bringer, 'Influence of Menopause on the Course of Diabetes Mellitus'. Clinique des Maladies Métaboliques et Endocriniennes, Hôpital St. Eloi, 34059 Montpellier Cedex 67, France

The following papers were read in Workshop sessions and the texts handed in to the congress Secretariate:

M. Albeaux-Fernet, 'Sodium Chloride and Menopause'. College of Medicine, Hôpital Laennec, Paris, France

J. J. Foldes, 'Hormonal *vs.* Non-hormonal Treatment of the Perimenopausal Complaints'. 12 Nehardea St., Tel-Aviv, Israel

M. Humphrey, 'The Empty Nest Syndrome: Theoretical Considerations'. Department of Psychiatry, St. George's Hospital Medical School, Clare House, Blackshaw Rd, London SW17, UK

K. Ichinoe, H. Yokota and N. Deguchi, 'On the Sexual Potentiality in the Hypothalamo–Pituitary Axis after the Reproductive Life Span'. Department of Obstetrics and Gynaecology, Wakayama Medical College, Japan 640

G. Krüskemper, M. Török and M. Berger, 'Menopause and Obesity: a Report of Psychological Data of 79 Women (Aged 40–59 Years) Taking Part in a Weight-Reduction Programme at a Medical Out-patient Clinic'. 2 Medizinische Klinik und Poliklinik, University of Düsseldorf, Düsseldorf, West Germany

G. Krüskemper, M. Török and H. Reidel, 'The Psychological Investigation (MMPI) of 59 Women Before and During the Menopause: a Follow-up after Five Years'. Address as above

M. Lévrier, 'Action du Moxestrol en Période de Ménopause'. 24, av de Lattre de Tassigny, 33400 Talence-Bordeaux, France

I. Mori, N. Takeda and T. Ikeda, 'Serum Gonadotrophin and its Response to the Administration of Gonadotrophin-Releasing Hormone in Normal Women with Ageing'. Department of Obstetrics and Gynaecology, Faculty of Medicine, Kagoshima University, Japan

G. Oelsner, D. Serr, A. Eshkol and B. Lunenfeld, 'The Early Menopause Syndrome in Secondary Amenorrhea'. The Chaim Sheba Medical Centre, Tel Hashomer, Tel Aviv University Medical School, Israel

U. Schalaster, 'Differences in Complaints about Health in Rural and Urban Women betwen 45 and 55 Years of Age'. Ulmenstrasse 10, 5309 Meckenheim-Merl, West Germany

L. Schubert, 'A Comparison of the Effects of Cyclophenil, Estradiol Valerianate and Placebo in Post-menopausal Women'. Via Friuli 51, 20135 Milan, Italy

S. Takenaka, I. Mori and Y. Tsuneyoshi, 'Steroid Hormones in the Blood of Women with Ageing—Particularly in the Climacteric Stage'. Department of Obstetrics and Gynaecology, Faculty of Medicine, Kagoshima University, Kagoshima, Japan

M. A. Weill-Hallé, 'Considerations about the Suggestion of the FDA Concerning Sequential Contraceptives: Possible Consequences for Estrogen Therapy in Women over Forty'. 77 av Paul Doumer, Paris 16e, France

List of Participants

T. Abe	Japan	D. Costes	France
Gullan Agerbak	Denmark	Françoise Couderc	France
M. Albeaux-Fernet	France	P. G. Crosignani	Italy
R. Alvart	France	G. H. Culpepper, Jr	USA
J. L. Ambrus	USA	W. Cyran	West Germany
N. Araki	Japan	S. Dalla Pria	Italy
D. J. Aravantinos	Greece	J. A. Davies	UK
A. Audebert	France	A. Deane	UK
R. J. Beard	UK	R. Demol	Belgium
E. L. Bellin	USA	J. Dequeker	Belgium
M. Ben-David	Israel	M. Detilleux	France
Irène Bernard	France	S. A. Duursma	The Netherlands
N. Bernassola	Italy	G. M. Edwards	The Netherlands
Catherine Blacker	France	A. E. G. Fanard	Belgium
D. G. T. Bloomer	UK	P. Fedor-Freybergh	Sweden
J.-L. Bodarwe	Belgium	Marcha Flint	USA
Lorraine Boykin	USA	J. J. Foldes	Israel
G. Braeken	Belgium	C. Forman	USA
P. C. Brand	UK	P. Fugere	Canada
J. H. Branolte	The Netherlands	R. F. Fuller	USA
G. Bryce	USA	Mirjam Furuhjelm	Sweden
J. C. Burch	USA	M. E. Gahwyler	USA
Nicole Burkel	France	R. D. Gambrell, Jr.	USA
L. Cammer	USA	U. Gaspard	Belgium
Simone Casabon	France	M. Gelinet	France
M. J. Casey	USA	S. Geller	France
J. C. Castanier	France	N. G. Georgecopoulos	Greece
L. W. Cellio	USA	G. S. Gordan	USA
S. K. Chakravarti	UK	F. H. Gottdiener	USA
A. C. Comninos	Greece	R. B. Greenblatt	USA
I. D. Cooke	UK	J. Grenier	France

Ilse Gretzmacher	West Germany	W. D. Odell	USA
J. P. Grison	France	A. Onnis	Italy
N. Guéritée	France	E. Oppenheim	USA
M. Harter	France	D. D. Oram	UK
G. A. Hauser	Switzerland	H. C. van Paassen	The Netherlands
J. Hazard	France	N. Parisis	Greece
E. Henderson	UK	J. Picazo	Spain
Kathryn Henderson	USA	S. Pino	USA
M. L'Hermite	Belgium	L. Poller	UK
D. G. Hertz	Israel	R. Punnonen	Finland
C. C. J. Höhner	The Netherlands	J. A. Queralt	USA
M. Humphrey	UK	L. Rauramo	Finland
H. Husslein	Austria	F. P. Rhoades	USA
K. Ichinoe	Japan	U. De Ridder	Belgium
T. Ikeda	Japan	C. Robyn	Belgium
L. Jaszmann	The Netherlands	J. E. Rodriguez-Soriano	Spain
Rachel Jenkins	USA	H. Rozenbaum	France
D. Kaskarelis	Greece	F. Ruggieri	Italy
P. A. van Keep	Belgium	Nancy G. Sandman	USA
P. Kemeter	Austria	G. Sansa	Italy
Suzanne Kepes	France	Ubrike Schalaster	West Germany
P. Kicovic	The Netherlands	E. Schleyer-Saunders	UK
R. M. Klapper	USA	G. T. Schneider	USA
H.-P. Klotz	France	L. Schubert	Italy
N. K. Kofinas	Greece	Helga Schützel	West Germany
H. Kopera	Austria	Martha H. de Sereday	Argentina
Gertude Krüskemper	West Germany	D. Serr	Israel
H. L. Krüskemper	West Germany	L. Severne	Belgium
U. Larsson-Cohn	Sweden	S. R. Slater	UK
Ch. Lauritzen	West Germany	S. Soihet	Peru
P. E. Lebech	Denmark	Joie Smith	USA
Christiane Lefebvre	France	C. Stoepker	The Netherlands
M. Lévrier	France	J. W. W. Studd	UK
T. H. C. Lewis	Canada	S. Takenaka	Japan
C. Longcope	USA	L. Tax	The Netherlands
C. E. Lyght	USA	J. Teter	Poland
M. M. Madlener	The Netherlands	A. Thénot	France
V. B. Mahesh	USA	J. H. H. Thijssen	The Netherlands
B. Maoz	Israel	D. Tomita	Japan
F. Marcelli	Italy	T. Ueda	Japan
D. Martin	USA	W. H. Utian	South Africa
S. Matsumoto	Japan	A. Vagogne	France
J. B. McKinlay	USA	G. Vanhulle	Belgium
S. M. McKinlay	USA ·	D. J. Vassilopoulos	Greece
J. Mirouze	France	E. Vázquez	Mexico
I. Mori	Japan	A. Vizzotto	Italy
Barbara Mühe	West Germany	G. Weiland	West Germany
J. P. Mumford	The Netherlands	Marie A. Weill-Hallé	France
S. Nagasako	Japan	W. E. Wellman	USA
A. Netter	France	R. Wenner	Switzerland
P. Nicolau	France	M. A. H. M. Wiegerinck	The Netherlands
E. Nishida	Japan	J. Wittebolle	Belgium
B. E. C. Nordin	UK	H. Yokota	Japan
M. Notelovitz	USA		

Index

Acknowledgements

The Congress was held under the auspices of the American Geriatric Society and the Medical Faculty of the University of Montpellier. Special thanks are due to Ayerst International for their generous support, both financial and consultative, and to the following:

Miles Laboratories, USA; Organon International, Holland; Upjohn, USA; Von Heyden GmbH, West Germany; and the Compagnie des Salins du Midi et des Salines de l'Est, France.